The 2 Hour Dental Start-up

Do you have the fire of an entrepreneur for a dental start-up?

The 2 Hour Dental Start-up is a seminar laying out the sequential process of opening a successful dental practice. You will gain knowledge from industry professionals such as; lenders, CPAs, realtors, attorneys, designers, and contractors walking you through their role in a dental start-up.

The 2 Hour
Dental Start-up

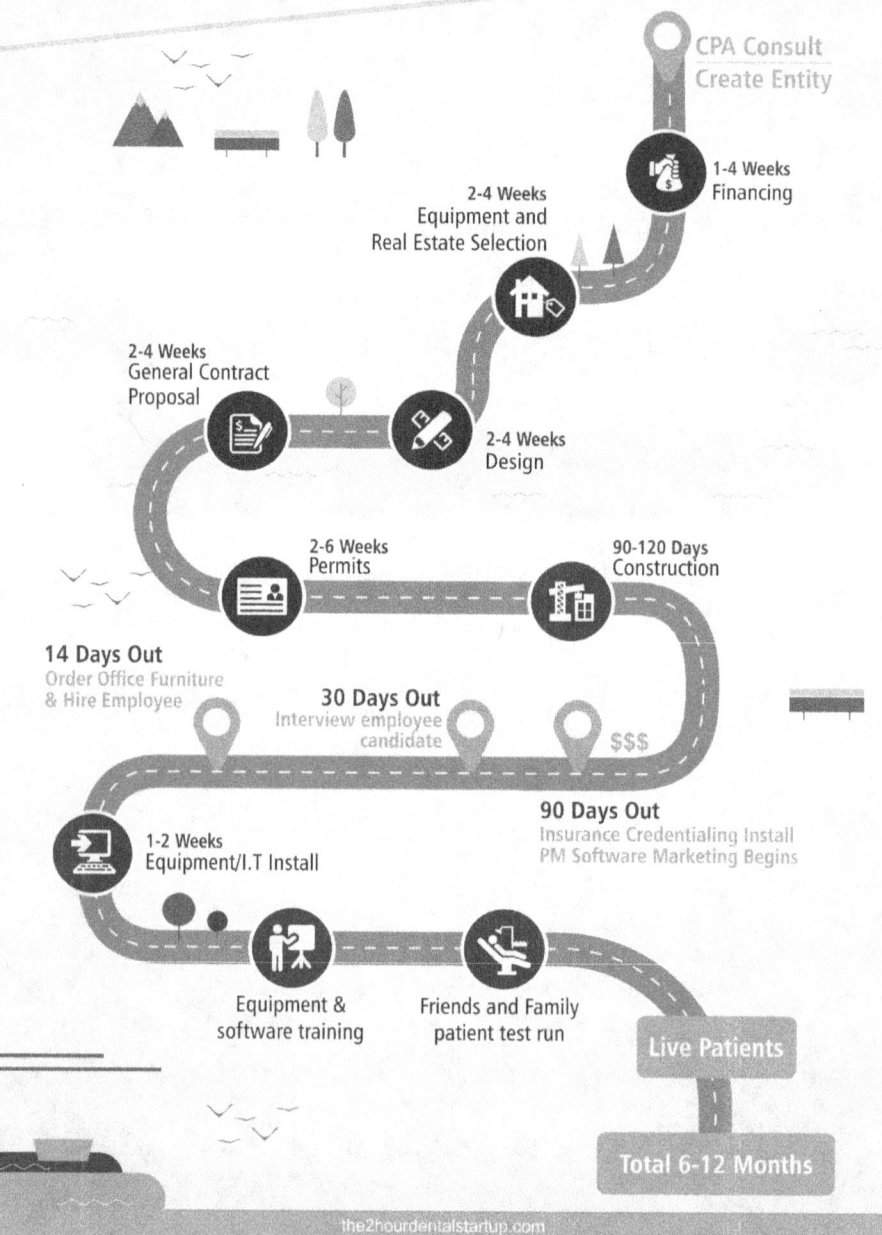

CPA Consult
Create Entity

1-4 Weeks
Financing

2-4 Weeks
Equipment and
Real Estate Selection

2-4 Weeks
General Contract
Proposal

2-4 Weeks
Design

2-6 Weeks
Permits

90-120 Days
Construction

14 Days Out
Order Office Furniture
& Hire Employee

30 Days Out
Interview employee
candidate

$$$

90 Days Out
Insurance Credentialing Install
PM Software Marketing Begins

1-2 Weeks
Equipment/I.T Install

Equipment &
software training

Friends and Family
patient test run

Live Patients

Total 6-12 Months

the2hourdentalstartup.com

2

Table of Contents

Acknowledgements

Thank you to all involved in producing this book. Your industry knowledge is valuable and well earned throughout the years of service. Thank you for each company's support and the employees that are the cornerstone to aid such a wonderful industry. And of course this book would not be in existence without the entrepreneur spirit of the independent dentist. Keep that alive.

Foreward

This book is for every dentist that wants to begin the venture of becoming an entrepreneur by starting their own dental practice from scratch. There is a sequence to this process that, if followed, will yield more positive results and less stress. Starting a practice has a beginning and an end, but there are many steps in the middle that parallel each other. Sometimes multiple decisions must be made and half the time these decisions are not related, such as; how long of a lease and what color upholstery to pick. There is a lot of time and money required during this endeavor. However if done correctly, it can be fun. Use this book as a guiding point in getting started. Each chapter was written by a professional that is proficient in their respective segment of the dental industry. We do this day in and day out and have assisted in an exuberant amount of dental start-ups. Good luck and enjoy the read.

Eric Swarvar
Dental Industry Extraordinaire

Chapter 1
Your Prepared Mindset
Clarity Focus Execute

By Eric Swarvar

On a chilly November morning in Texas, my associate Richard and I were waiting at a Starbucks for a dentist to arrive. This dentist was trained in South Korea, but attended a condensed program in the United States to be licensed as a practicing dentist. After a few years in private practice, he decided to begin the journey of a dental start-up. Through our conversation I was using substratal terms such as; LOI, shell space, NNN, finish-out, and TI allowance. It was apparent he did not understand. I asked two simple questions, "What is your time frame? Where are you building?" To this day his response blows me away. He pointed to a dirt lot across the street and said, he was "going in, in 6 weeks". A dirt lot is 12 months from construction to opening as a dental office with many variables working in the favor of the builder. Time after time, I have been involved in many meetings that are similar to this situation. Not all are this conspicuous, however it confirms; dentist DENTAL*, and everything else is trivial. Thus, the 2 Hour Dental Start-up seminars were born.

I have always understood that dentists are clinicians first. Beyond that there are several other roles we will discuss later that must be portrayed. But no dentist has construction manager as a common job title. Even if you are familiar with the other roles of starting a dental practice. From securing lending to real estate negotiator, certified public accountant, insurance credential specialist, architect, dental equipment specialist, information technology specialist, marketer, and human resource manager. These are just some of the titles needed to start your own dental practice. For the purpose of this book I am focusing on:
• Securing financing
• Location selection
• Accounting as a business plan
• Dental office design and the process of construction
• Equipment selection - operatory design
• Marketing, its not just advertising
• Human Resource as a business strategy

*DENTAL as a verb, the act of clinical dentistry.

The information contained in this book is from accumulated experiences of hundreds of dental start-ups as seen from the professionals within the industry. I have seen successful and mediocre start-ups with a few failures. I am removing my sales hat to offer this guidance to give back to the industry I love. My goal is to provide a systemic approach and limit the stress of doing a successful dental start-up.

If you think that this process is easy, stop reading, give this book to a friend and become a career associate. Opening a dental practice takes sacrifice, hard work, and chutzpah. All this is needed just to open the doors. This process takes a present conscious mind, the willingness to learn, lead, and trust business advisors.

Congratulations if you are still reading. It is imperative that you define your terms of success. Do not turn to social media or your peers to seek out what this achievement looks like. A successful practice in one part of the country is not the same for the other. I have read so many obstinate statements of glory on social media that are implausible to apply as a standard for a business. Set your own standards and goals.
Before you can execute any major undertaking, you should have a vision and before you have a vision, you should have clarity for your project. A clear mind is a focused mind. Clarity, vision, execution! Clarity, vision, execution!

To gain clarity in owning a dental practice, revisit an old question and ask a few new. Why did you become a dentist? This is a question that is ambiguously subjective and can loose its will with every passing day. Think back to when you decided to be a dentist Are you fulfilling your vision that you had of yourself in dental school? If not, how have you strayed and is it for the better or worse?

What are your personal goals? What are your professional goals? Your professional goals need to serve your personal goals. When you decide to start your own business, goals have to be sacrificed in the short term to meet your longterm ambitions. However the more personal goals you sacrifice, your ambitious mindset will deteriorate. Are you willing to sacrifice finances, time, and some relationships?

If you are planning a dental start-up, don't:

- Plan a wedding
- Plan a divorce
- Get pregnant
- Probate a will
- Build a house
- Move
- Buy a sports car
- Buy a second home
- Quit your associateship
- Pick up sky diving
- Downhill mountain biking
- Climb Mt. Everest.

In other words, do not make a decision you can't unwind. The above are major life decisions and should wait until you are positive cashflow on your business.

All goals need to be written down. If you do not write out your goals, they are just a thought. A thought can easily become a moving target and you will compromise your vision just to make yourself feel better. Always write down and display your objectives and evaluate them. It is important to have daily, monthly, yearly, and BHAG (big hairy audacious goals) generally a 10+ year goal. Review each goal with the equivalent time set, except the BHAG; review that daily.
What is your vision of ownership?

- Be your own boss
- Control your own schedule

- Build equity in a business through time (wealth building strategy)
- Create a higher income opportunity than an associate position
- Build wealth by being a business owner
- Freedom and flexibility in ownership
- Practice freely from corporate oversight
- Become an elite clinician
- Own multiple practices
- Land owner, landlord, or developer
- Create high income and be complacent

There are only two types of dental practices left in America: community based practices and competitive market practices.

Community based dental practices are located where dental services are needed. Generally in a rural location, less population density, and underserved by not just dentist but other services like medical and retail. Community based practices are generally in a lower income population with less access to healthcare. The rent or land cost are typically less than an urban/suburban setting. The average employment wage is typically less and with less employers, there are less jobs, which drives down wages in these markets. Since there are less jobs employees tend to be more loyal. As a business you can keep limited hours because there is less competition. Since there is less competition the marketing budget can be significantly less. Most of these dental practices are typically pain driven with mixed payment from PPO insurances, cash paying patients, and Medicaid. There are less specialists in the area which will allow the general dentist to do their choice of procedures. The general dentist performing specialty services such as; endodontics, placement of implants, soft tissue surgery, and orthodontics, will not be frowned upon by specialists. Dentist in these markets typically can be major community investors or leaders.

Competitive market practice is based in an urban and sub-urban community with a high population density and a saturation of dentist to populous. These practices need to leverage every medium of marketing to carve out their niche in a market that already has copious access to dental care. These markets are generally in a higher income population with employers offering benefits such as dental insurance. There is an abundance of healthcare and dental providers. This opulence of dental practices means a high level of competition, which means the practice owner must have a high marketing budget. Because of the nature of these markets, there is a higher level of expectation for technology increasing the investment in equipment. The presence of other industries give way to pre-eminent competition for quality employees meaning payroll is higher and loyalty is lower. The patients and workforce are typically more educated. In order to be available to your obstinate base the practice should work expanded hours and some Fridays or Saturdays. Most of these markets have plenty of specialists which discourage from performing expanded procedures. Other peer dentist will look at you as competition. Generally dentist in these markets do not live in the community the practice is in and that is acceptable.

Build Your Team of Advisors

Once clarity is established it is time to build your team of trusted advisors. Trust is the foundation of all positive relationships. This conjunction is bilateral and driven by communication. Just like a dental practice is a business designed to generate a profit, no one is going to take on a client if it is not a benefit to them. Fair market value for goods and services is important, however if you marginalize these partners down to the dime their incentive to work on your behalf is abated. Just like in dental work, cheap is cheap.

The financial lender is equipped to administer all relationships and assist keeping the project on time. The lender is the conductor of the network and can introduce you to trusted vendors.

Real estate representatives are paid by the landowner. An accomplished agent will assist in researching a favorable location and negotiate on your behalf to get the best rent and tenant improvement allowance (T&I).

The appropriate dental equipment company (DEC) can consult on designing the office layout based on input from the dentist and experience from the designer. The DEC can assist in site checks during the construction phase of the project. This is important to ensure the mechanical, electrical, and plumbing for the dental equipment is duly located during construction. This invaluable service should be considered in the price of the equipment.

A quality CPA firm is familiar with the intricacies of running a dental practice as a business and is the dentist's closest confidant on the business side of dentistry during their career.

A general contractor (GC) is only as good as the subcontractors they use. The subcontractors know how a GC builds their reputation. It is not necessary to select a GC that is specific to building dental spaces but it is important. It is also significantly helpful if the lender, DEC, or real estate broker is familiar with the GC you are using.

Since electronic health records (EHR) are the standard in dentistry and the dentist must comply with HIPPA regulations, selecting a medical/dental information technology company to partner with and manage your network is key. This is a relationship the dentist should consider long-term. Ransomware is a real problem for small businesses, and the appropriate maintenance and security should take place.

Human resource (HR) is generally an after thought for most and associated with firing an employee. However, HR should be a strategy to build and scale your practice with the appropriate human capital. Outsourcing HR has become affordable and is important to build the team you desire.

Butts in chairs are what drives revenue. Despite the style of practice you choose, you need to let people know you are open for business. Collaborating with a marketing firm that meets your needs is important. Marketing tends to get overlooked and dismissed by many small businesses. Do not make this mistake. Having a website, mailers, and a sign hung is not marketing. Marketing is an ongoing effort involving the full scope of business. From production to selling goods, greeting a phone call to dismissing the patient, soft skills should be taught and reviewed with team members to create the type of environment you desire. These are the subtleties that build brands. Mark Cuban said it best, "Marketing dollars do not build brands. Product satisfaction and execution does."

Items to marginalize are transitional based purchases such as; your sign company, office furniture, office decor, phone service, internet, and pm software. These items will be purchased with very little need for service after the transition has occurred. This is a small subset of the cost of a dental start-up, however it can add up.

This process should be an exciting and enjoyable venture. Two weeks before opening and the first two weeks after are always the most stressful. Do not schedule a hard date for an open house or a ribbon cutting during this time. I can assure you the odds are not in your favor to hit the target date. If you desire an open house or grand opening, schedule this event 2-3 months after your soft opening. This will allow you to work out any flaws, create a positive patient experience, and begin to create a working relationship with your team.

In the upcoming chapters a systemic approach will be defined by industry experts responsible for hundreds of dental start-ups. This approach is a guide to opening a successful dental practice from scratch.

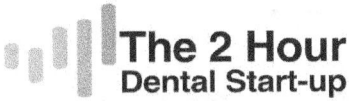

The 2 Hour
Dental Start-up

CLARITY | FOCUS | EXECUTE

1. PERSONAL **GOALS**

2. PROFESSIONAL **GOALS**

3. WHY DID YOU BECOME **A DENTIST?**

4. WHY DO YOU WANT TO DO **A START-UP?**

5. VISION FOR YOUR **START-UP!**

Chapter 2

Preparing for your Lender

By Jennifer Edwards

You have dreamed about starting your own practice since day one of dental school. You are so close to graduation you can taste it. How do you prepare to open your own business, specifically a dental practice?

Preplanning

Pre-work:

- Associate a minimum of two years to educate yourself on how a practice runs, drives business, collects money, and manages a schedule

  o Learn what you DON'T want to do in your practice

- SAVE, SAVE, SAVE

  o Every dentist's instinct is paying down student loan debt immediately - **resist the urge**

  o Building personal cash reserves

- Know your credit score - 720 or higher is preferred

These are tips I wish I could share with every dental student in their third to fourth year of dental school. Upon graduation, you will most likely have student loan debt and that is OK. Lending institutions do not penalize you for having student loan debt. Dentists tend to be debt adverse, because their first instinct is to start paying down student loans aggressively while working as an associate. **Do not do that**. Keep your loan current, make the payments, and meet your obligations. But build liquidity. **Cash, cash, cash.** Put cash in the bank. More is better. There is no formula. It does not need to be 10 percent or 30 percent of the loan you are trying to get, but more is better. When you get ready to start a business you need to have a cushion for your personal life. Cash on hand will prepare you to help pay the mortgage, feed the dog and buy clothes for the kids when income drops. You still need to be able to live a life while starting a business. And until the business is profitable, which can take anywhere from two to five years, your personal life should not starve financially. If you have a pretty good cash cushion, lenders feel more comfortable that you can manage cash. Do not get overwhelmed paying off your student loan debt.

Don't make a financial decision you cannot unwind, such as buy a big house or purchase a fancy new car. You're finally out of school making some decent money. If you're working as an associate you're probably working really hard and wanting to having some fun is a natural idea. But if your dream is owner-ship, do yourself a favor and keep your debt load low. Those things will come but be conservative until you realize your dream of ownership. Then you can start planning for those things.

Know your credit score. There are several free websites where you can get an idea of your credit score. Most major credit cards offer some type of credit score service for free. Know what is on your credit before you apply for credit. Uncover any past scrupulous judgements against you such as; when you were in college, that one apartment you broke the lease on and they filed a judgment against you. This happens all too often and can put you in a bind when you are trying to qualify for financing. Or if there is a medical collection because you went to the doctor while you were in college and they never sent you a bill. Now you owe thirty-eight dollars to the E.R. Be informed, resolve, and be aware of what your score is. A minimum score of 720 is recommended, but higher is better.

The Hard Work

- Develop a business plan

- o Why should patients choose you as their dentist?

- o What will you offer?

- o Fee for Service or In Network

- o Budget to start-up
    - Finish Out/Construction
    - Equipment
    - Working Capital
    - # of employees

- o Include three years of financial projections - your CPA can assist

- Understand what it takes to get financing in place

  - o Prepare a COMPLETE financial package

  - o See Exhibit for list of most requested financial information

- Select your lender

  - o Do they have a specialty or understanding of your profession?

    - Do they speak **Dentist**?

Develop a business plan and have an idea of how your practice will be successful. What can you bring to the table as an individual that makes you unique in your market place? Put your vision on paper. If your vision is not written it is difficult to hold yourself to it. This can be difficult to lay out in print. However, you want to borrow anywhere from five hundred to a million dollars depending on many variables. You need to have a plan and you need to be able to articulate that plan to your lender. A year or two years before starting this process, start formulating your vision for your practice. What is your competitive advantage? The best time to do this is when working as an associate, because you know the successes and shortcomings of those practices. Write those things down. Knowing what you do not want to do is as important as knowing what you want to do.

About three years ago, I had a dentist come to me with a full blown PowerPoint presentation. He not only had his technical stuff in there, He also knew how much he needed to borrow, what he was going to spend it on and what needed to happen in the practice in terms of daily production to break even and make a profit. He was telling me his vision, selling me his brand, and had put a significant amount of thought into why he wanted his own practice and why it was going to be successful. He had so much passion and belief in what he was going to do. By the way, I should tell you, he opened his practice and he is killing it. His patients love him. His employees love him. He translated his passion for what he does into that presentation and was able to realize his dream of ownership because he visualized it so well. He is driving a healthy practice from it. He put it on paper and believed in it. He could sell his passion. Today he is still selling it. He is having to adjust his plan. COVID impacted him as it did everybody. But because he had a plan, he was able to get back on track and be true to his original purpose because he had really committed himself in the beginning.

Dentists tell me all of the time, "Business is not my forte" or "I didn't take any business classes" or "They didn't teach me that at dental school". Another reason I was impressed (and this is something we hear a lot), dentists are not businesspeople. They are scientists and medical professionals who treat humans. If you plan to own your own office, do the work to make it successful. Surround yourself with trusted advisors, do the research, build a plan. This is one of the biggest commitments you will ever make in your life. It can be one of the most rewarding journeys as well. Build yourself a road map and plan to be successful in building your legacy. You will thank yourself later down the road.

The business plan has been written. You have cash in the bank and your credit score is 720 or higher. Now it is time to select your lender.

A few things to consider:

- Does the lender offer Dental Specific Financing?
- Does your Banker speak "Dentist"?

Many banks/lenders have specific financing available for dentists looking to start a practice. The average general dentistry practice takes $500,000 - $750,000 for a start-up. This includes: finish out of lease space, equipment, and working capital. Pre-COVID, there were a number of programs in the marketplace that offered 100% financing for dental start-ups. The Pandemic has impacted what most lenders are offering today. Common programs offer 80-85% financing with a required equity (cash) injection of 15-20%. This means if your start-up budget is $500,000 the bank would provide 80% financing or a loan for $400,000 and you would contribute $100,000. Most lenders offer conventional financing with a fixed rate and a term of up to 10 years. They will include interest only draw periods so that you can advance on the loan as the project progresses.

Most lenders will require an assignment of life insurance in the amount of the loan on the doctor. Malpractice Insurance and Disability Insurance will also need to be in place at the time of the loan closing. Addressing those issues prior to application can save you a lot of stress.

Focus on lenders familiar with dentistry and those that offer dental specific financing. Your CPA, Dental Equipment Specialist, and contractor will usually know the banks that are lending in your area. Ask them for referrals or an introduction. Good people work with good people and are willing to introduce you to those that can assist in achieving your goal.

FINANCIAL NEEDS LIST
FOR A START-UP LOAN

01. 3 years personal tax returns for all guarantors
02. 3 years business tax returns for all existing businesses
03. Personal Financial Statement
04. Bank Statements (personal for liquidity verification)
05. Debt Schedule (if applicable)
06. Year to Date Balance Sheet and Income Statement for all existing businesses (if applicable)
07. Proof of Insurance:
08. Malpractice
09. Disability
10. Life Insurance
11. Hazard (when available)
12. Copy of Driver's License for all Guarantors
13. Name and Tax ID of Borrowing Entity (if formed)
14. Secretary of State Documents
15. IRS EIN letter (if available)
16. Operating Agreement (Draft)
17. Resume for all guarantors
18. Business Plan
19. 3 years of revenue projections
20. Copy of lease (if available) or LOI
21. Budget/Use of proceeds/equipment quotes

The 2 Hour
Dental Start-up

Chapter 3

Real Estate Exploration, Preparation, and Execution

By Peter Hays

"Dr. Williams? Good evening, this is Peter Hays with Practice Real Estate Group. Your lender asked that we touch base regarding your dental startup? Our firm specializes in real estate for dentists and group practices. We help you decide where to open in a market, locate and evaluate the best lease & purchase options in that area, provide Dentist to Population Ratio studies & demographic reports, negotiate the contract and manage all parties from start to finish. What day is good for you to grab coffee?"

Our scheduled meeting comes around and I wait for a husband and wife at a local coffee shop. The couple met in dental school and have since worked as associates at the same national chain for the past 3 years. Lenders are happy to finance a practice for a husband-and-wife team assuming financials are reasonable, a sign of a serious future business owner is having an idea of your ability to finance a business and also provides your team (the dentist and their real estate broker) a general reference as to what you can realistically lease or purchase. After explaining the process from initial meeting to Grand Opening, and quickly reviewing some of the terms we would be pushing for in the Letter of Intent (items like Construction Period and Lease Commencement Date, Operating Expenses, SNDA, CAM caps), it became clear that they are new to the commercial real estate world. Dentistry is hard and real estate is new to you, there will be a lot of unfamiliar terms and processes throughout a project like this and your team will be there to answer any questions you have. So, how do you get from a Cafe Latte to an open dental practice? Let's break the process down into three phases: (1) Exploration, (2) Preparation, and (3) Execution. Naturally, we begin at Exploration.

Exploration

This stage is where you start laying out your business model at 20,000 feet. Part of the point of an initial meeting is for a proper introduction, and coffee of your choice, but our main goal here is to identify points of concern and drivers that will eventually lead us to defining an area for a Market Study. We will get into what a "Market Study" is later in this discussion.

The initial question to the husband and wife was "Why do you want to open your own practice?". That's a fairly broad and open-ended question, the goal here is to think about what pains are causing you to want to get out of your current situation and into ownership. Their answer was simple, the drive from their house was too far and they wanted flexibility. We have a breakthrough. "What is a reasonable drive time for you from your house, 30 minutes is an hour you will be in your car every day, is that too long?". They were fine with a 20-minute drive time each way. "Do you have a non-compete at your current practice?". They did, a ten-mile radius from the office. That non-compete radius is not uncommon. "What type of practice are you hoping to open? Medicaid, PPO, FFS?". Let's briefly review each:

Medicaid: Government Subsidized Healthcare – Typically located in low to middle class neighborhoods. These offices bill to the government's Medicaid/CHIP programs at a lower margin than PPO and Fee for Service. Overhead will have to be lower than other practices, and your patient volume will be higher.

PPO: Preferred Provider Organization – Your clientele will pay mostly through their insurance plans. Other expenses not explicitly covered through their plans will be billed to them. These office's demographics can be a mix of lower, middle and upper classes, depending on the health care plans offered by local businesses.

Fee for Service: Cash Based Office – Typically the most expensive and will be located in pockets of the upper middle class and above. These clients will be paying for all services out of pocket. Be sure that your location supports this type of practice, and that you are prepared to handle the positives and negatives of each.

The Williams wanted to have a practice focused primarily towards PPO with some Medicaid. Eric asked in the opening of this book, "what is your timeframe?". This is an important question and can drive where you open as well. In this case, the timeline was flexible and they wanted to be in whichever project offered the best overall chance of success. Something we run into a lot when searching for a new location to place a startup or group is a lack of infrastructure. This is especially true in more rural and developing or growing markets. You can't lease what doesn't exist, but you can lease a project in the planning phase, or 1-2 years out. If you're hoping to open your doors as soon as possible, immediately, these "proposed" projects won't be a fit unless they are scheduled to deliver within a couple months. If there is more flexibility surrounding when you would like to be open, perhaps a proposed property would work for you. The timeframe I like to give and we find is applicable to most startups is 8-12 months from initial conversations with lenders and your real estate team to your Grand Opening. Below is a fairly conservative timeline assuming the building you wish to lease exists:

- 1 month to get financials to the bank.
- 1-2 months to locate an appropriate site.
- 1-2 months to negotiate an LOI on said site.
- 1-2 months to negotiate a lease or purchase agreement.
- 6 months to design, permit and construct space.

If you plan on purchasing a building, add 1-4 months for feasibility, title review and closing. Build out of the interior will take a similar amount of time, around 6 months. For ground up projects, plan for a minimum of 12 months for your project delivery and more realistically, 18 months. It's typical for land to be under contract for 6 months before closing, the building can take another 6-8 months to deliver and the build out of your space will be close to 6 months. Your long-term goals should be taken into consideration when you are deciding whether to lease or purchase. For those dentists that want to open a few locations annually, it's often a better business decision to lease. The asset requirement for a ground up is large and can equate to 3+ practices. If you would like to own one or two locations, purchasing a building or doing a ground up makes more sense. The path you take depends on the end goal.

With financing started, we have a general budget in place. Lenders will usually require a startup stay below a certain monthly rent number dependent on review of financials, which is a combination of the size of the space and the base rate. "Would you prefer an office or retail setting?". Retail is becoming more popular for medical and especially dental, but with retail and visibility, comes higher rents. If you prefer an office setting, you are usually able to lease a larger space because of the lower rental rates for these types of projects. A retail setting will typically require you take a bit smaller space to hit the lenders underwriting requirements. $7,500/Month is a popular number lenders will require you stay at or below for a first general dentistry practice.

Asking yourself a few simple questions like the ones above can help narrow down where you want to practice. We get the "Where is the best market, City, State to open?" question a lot. *There is opportunity everywhere, quality of life is important.* Taking the points that were negatively affecting the Williams quality of life, we were able to identify that the area they wanted to open their startup would be within a 20-minute drive time from their home, with area incomes of around $45,000-$80,000, with a portion of the area within their drive time being unavailable because of the non-compete with their current employer.

We now have actionable items, it's time to prepare and execute.

Preparation:

"It was great to meet you in person. I'll have our demographics team start the Market Study for the area we identified ASAP. I look forward to the opportunity to help with your project and we're confident you will find our processes and data useful.".

From this side of the table, I see two excited doctors that are understandably nervous about the upcoming adventure. These next couple months will require a lot of trust and attention, but it's the most exciting time for a startup. The point of the Preparation phase is to get you to the Execution phase, where you will execute a lease and begin construction. The Preparation phase includes the following steps:

1. Market Study
2. Property Report
3. Dentist to Population Ratio Study
4. Letter of Intent
5. Lease Negotiation

During the Preparation phase, it's important that you begin building your team around you. Before you have a contract ready to execute, you will want to have had discussions with the following industries and identified who you will be working with. Your broker will have recommendations and should make those introductions at the right time, which we will touch on in the appropriate sections below. Your team will include:

1. Lender
2. Contractor
3. Architect
4. Equipment Representative
5. Insurance Specialist
6. Real Estate Attorney
7. IT
8. Sign Company

What is a "Market Study" anyway? A Market Study is a step in the process that locates underserved areas prior to searching for sites in a market and running a site-specific Dentist to Population Ratio Study. We find this saves everyone involved time, no one enjoys getting excited about a project to find out there is too much competition and the bank won't approve the loan. For the Williams, we decided that a reasonable area for the couple to open their practice was within 20 minutes from their home, should have a blue-collar income and could not be within a 10 miles radius of their current employer. The area for the Market Study was around 38 square miles. We were able to identify 2 areas within the Market Study that had the incomes we were looking for, was outside of the non-compete and had a higher Dentist to Population Ratio than the rest of the areas in the study. Whether this is your first practice or 100th location, this is always a first step when narrowing down a market because it saves time.

Financing - The bank will be requesting financial information at this point, you will want to provide them with the requested information as soon as possible.

We have two areas now with similar demographics and competition from a high-level view, it's time to find property to lease. It should go without saying that the Property Report step is one of the most important parts of the project and process. "Location, Location, Location". The commercial real estate listing database is a bit more outdated and inaccurate than residential sites most people are used to using. It's suggested that your broker go through and call each location within the area decided on, verify the information and provide you with only the options that work. Something as simple as identifying office vs retail, current exclusives among current tenants and space available in the center should shorten the list from 75-100 properties to 10-20 real options, depending on the market. Reviewing an updated and verified list of properties does a couple things. First and foremost, the options you look at will be real options, something you can actually lease. Secondly and as equally important, you will have a better idea what the rates and operating expenses are of different quality sites. It's important for you to be as educated on the market as your real estate broker.

Contractor & Architect - It's a good time to start discussions with contractors and/or architects once you have properties in front of you. There are a couple ways to go about building your space. Some people prefer to hire an architect and bid out the plans to contractors, others prefer a contractor that will handle the entire thing. Your equipment rep may become involved in the design of the space and will work with either the architect, contractor or both. I highly suggested getting a contractor or architect into the space(s) you are interested in as soon as possible for an initial walkthrough. This walkthrough is an opportunity for discovery, our goal is to find anything that may add costs to the project before going to lease for leverage reasons. An equipment rep may also want to get into the space for similar reasons.

The Property Report for the two areas we looked into from the initial Market Study returned 15 properties that fit our size requirement, need for a retail setting and allowed general dentistry services. What qualities make a good location?

Visibility - Startups need all the visibility they can get, it's a simple form of free advertising. Hard corners, spaces fronting high traffic roads, lighted Intersections or next to high traffic tenants. Startup dentists benefit from high traffic environments such as Target, Walmart and HEB shopping centers. Other high traffic tenants such as Starbucks or Chipotle offer large crowds as well. If there are no available spaces in these types of centers, look for options that are near or adjacent to these types of centers.

New Construction - This isn't a necessity, however higher quality, newer centers are a common target for dental tenants looking for their first space. Most want to match the interior with the exterior with quality materials and looks.

Stand Alone Buildings - Sites in high traffic areas that stand by themselves are good targets for dental sites. Previously occupied restaurants, banks and anything located on hard corners or that front the roads provide good visibility.

Ease of Access - Patients need to be able to easily find and access the property. As an example, it may not be ideal to put your client on a highway where the entrance to the project is not easily identifiable and they must do a turn around to look for it again. Patients want to get in and out quickly, so this can be very important to your client.

Parking - It is important to understand your clients' needs when it comes to parking. Make sure there are no tenants that will take all of the parking, leaving patients having to walk a long distance or not be able to find a parking spot.

Signage - The bigger the facade, the more space for your building signage and visibility to passersby. If your building is a bit deeper than average, note that your signage area (facade) will be less and vice versa.

Of the 15 properties that were shortlisted at a high level, 4 properties had additional characteristics we want to see and offered similar visibility, contents, anchors and traffic flow. The Williams were excited about their options as they appeared on face value, but the more data to assist with a decision this big the better. After running a site-specific Dentist to Population Ratio Study for each of the 4 locations, we were able to identify one property that had a competition ratio that was reasonable enough to create elevated interest in that site over the other alternatives.

It's time to negotiate terms for a large and long-term contract. While rent and Tenant Improvement amounts are the main focus for new practice owners, the real purpose of a Letter of Intent is to limit risk as much as possible for yourself. It's important to keep in mind that this is true for the Landlord and their team as well, and compromises will have to come from both sides. So how do you get negotiations started? There are two options. Either you and your real estate broker submit a proposal to the Landlords team or the Landlord and their broker submit one to you. In the Williams case and as a regular practice, we prefer to submit our own Letter of Intent to the Landlord. We find our proposals are more comprehensive than most Landlords and contain about 30 terms specific to dental that we have identified as important over the last 10 years. The Landlord will sometimes want to use their standard form. Expect their standard form to be void of a lot of important information like renewal periods, relocation clauses, CAM caps, assignment rights, exclusive clauses. If a term is not covered while negotiating a Letter of Intent, it benefits the Landlord when you get to lease negotiations. Make sure any terms that you wish to include in a document originated by a Landlord are inserted prior to moving to lease negotiations.

Contractor & Architect - The further along you get in the Letter of Intent negotiations, the more the need becomes to have your contractor or architect do a walkthrough of the space. It's a lot easier to negotiate a few dollars more in Tenant Improvement Allowance now if you do find something, rather than at lease negotiations. Your equipment rep may also want to visit the site to check for things like support beams if they are assisting in the design of the space.

Frequently Asked Questions

1. What's a **Letter of Intent**? A LOI is a non-binding agreement between a Tenant and Landlord outlining terms of an agreement. This is not a legally binding document, however, is used in good faith by both parties to decide larger terms prior to involving attorneys. Not negotiating a LOI prior to drafting a lease creates additional attorney fees and increased costs.

2. Can I assign my Lease? Yes, this should be negotiated prior to finalizing the LOI. It's important to be relieved of obligations should you decide to sell your practice in the future.

3. Should I create a business entity for my practice? The creation of a business entity for your practice shields you from personal liability in the case of a lawsuit against your practice. The business entity acts as a shield that protects your personal assets like your car or house. In the event of damages being awarded against your practice, a court may rule that your personal assets be seized to satisfy the award if your business assets are not enough to cover the entire amount. Creating a business entity means that a plaintiff cannot recover against any assets outside of the business entity. In other words, the plaintiff can only recover against property your business entity and its affiliates (depending on the type of entity) own, and not against property that is owned in your name. This is one of the most basic premises of business law but is nonetheless a very important one.

4. Do the Operating Expenses Increase? One of the facts of being a Tenant is that costs will increase from year to year. This is because of increased costs to your Landlord due either to inflation or increased one-time expenditures impacting the property. Each year, the Landlord will provide you

with an estimate for the next year's operating expenses. Depending on the accuracy of that estimate, you may be owed money, or you may be required to pay additional monies, so long as they do not exceed the cap. Remember, you share is proportional to the amount of space you are leasing as compared to the entire building, and not just portions that are currently occupied by other tenants.

5. What is Tenant Construction Allowance - The Tenant Construction Allowance is a dollar amount per square foot that a Landlord will provide to a new Tenant. The idea is to use this money on the costs associated building out the inside of your new office. With the help of a contractor, space planner, or architect, you will design the layout of your new office to meet your specific requirements. The landlord provides this amount based on 1) the current condition of the space, 2) the expected length of the lease term (typically 10 years for medical tenants), and 3) an assumption of good credit.

6. What is an exclusive clause? Exclusivity clauses protect tenants from direct competitors moving into spaces in the same retail project or office building. The Landlord agrees not to lease space to future tenants who provide the same services as you and warrants that there are currently no other tenants providing the same services. This right gives tenants a reassurance regarding competition in the area, and an expectation of the service not being oversupplied in the demographic market. Ideally, an exclusive clause gives the Tenant a monopoly on the type of service or good they sell within the retail shopping center or office building.

7. Do I need to address signage in the LOI? A tenant's right to signage space is crucial for location identification and marketing reasons. Being able to put a panel on a pylon or monument or have store-

front signage helps customers locate your new practice within a retail center. Further, having larger storefront signage, particularly if facing a busy street, is an advertisement in itself. Knowing how much signage available and what type of signage will be will help you acquire the services of a sign installer. You will want this type of service scheduled for completion during the Tenant Construction Period, and you will want your sign service provider to review the lease before execution to make sure the signage terms are agreeable and doable in your budget. If you need help locating a sign service provider, we can help.

8. What's an SNDA? This stands for Subordination, Non-Disturbance and Attornment. The main point of this term is to protect your right to lease should something happen with the Landlord, like they sell to another party or file for bankruptcy.

After about a month and 5-6 rounds of negotiations between our team and the Landlord, the Williams and I are happy with where we sit term wise in the Letter of Intent. TI Allowance is a reasonable percentage of the overall rent paid, and there were smaller wins throughout the remainder of the proposal. The next step here involves executing the LOI and having the Landlord's attorney draft a contract. You will need an attorney, specifically a real estate attorney, to review the terms that were agreed to in the LOI. We want to make sure the language was interpreted correctly in the draft and it favors us over the Landlord, if the language was meant to in the LOI. This process will take a month or two until an executable contract is ready for both parties to sign.

Financing - Most lenders that have a specialized practice finance arm will require a lease draft before they can fully approve a loan. The LOI will have most of the information they need, like rates, TI allowances, abated rent periods, to give general approval of the loan, but it's usually not official until they have a copy of the Lease.

Contractor/Architect - It's important to have your contractor or architect review any construction, Landlord or Tenant work exhibits. This will keep otherwise hidden costs out of your project. Additionally, to hit your target opening, using the Lease negotiation period to finalize designs help assure you are ready to permit the day following lease execution or delivery of your space.

Insurance Specialists - There is a section of the Lease that will outline insurance policies a Tenant is required to keep. We suggest sending that portion of the Lease to the insurance specialist to make sure what is requested is market, and doesn't substantially alter any current insurance policies you have. Common insurance policies required when leasing include disability, life, office overhead, homeowners, and liability.

Sign Company - Prior to executing a Lease, have your signage company review the Landlords signage requirements and provide a rendering for approval. This rendering will be inserted into the Lease as an exhibit.

Execution

We have reached a major point of action, Lease execution. You have been approved for financing. You know what type of practice you will be operating. Your location has been selected. Contractors, architects and insurance specialists have reviewed their sections of the contract. Plans are ready to be submitted for permitting. Equipment may have been selected at this point, payment pending financing. Insurance has been purchased. Time to execute the contract and make this project a reality.

The execution phase consists of everything needed to go from a shell space, or demoing a current build out, to a working, thriving office. You are 5-7 months into this process and are ready to go back to doing what you enjoy, practicing dentistry. What are you missing?

1. A website was once considered a value-add feature, is now a necessity in the dental world. Websites to promote, or at least simply confirm your practice's existence are expected. Websites are especially important for the more affluent demographics. Your clients hope to be able to research you, your staff, and the services you offer. A website will be your opportunity to showcase your practice to a perspective client. Website design should begin as soon as you know the address of your new office and you can support the marketing of the website. Important aspects of your websites design and function include: Site Longevity, Keywords, Content/Relevance, Webpage Optimization ("Meta-Tags"), Inbound Links.

2. Credentialing can be a long, strenuous process if not approach systematically. If credentialing is a part of your practice's business plan, it is a necessary evil. Credentialing is the process of reaching out to appropriate insurance companies who represent your client demographics and going through their vetting process. This process usually includes request of financials from your office.

3. Your staff will be the backbone of your new office. As a small operation, you may choose to forgo hiring anything more than a receptionist and part-time hygienist to begin with. As your practice grow, staffing will be one of your largest, if not the largest line-item expenses on the expense report. More importantly, your receptionist and assistants will be the face and voice of your practice. There are many staffing agencies that cater to dentists. There are other online routes or word of mouth referrals to recruit quality talent. Do not take this step lightly, as it will set the tone of your day in day out operations. Hiring

should begin a few months before you open your doors. If possible, have a dry run with family and friends where your new staff has a chance to run through what a daily operation will look like.

4. IT, Hardware and Software can all be purchased through a multitude of dealers. Consult a salesman who has experience with dental practice management. Your required computer hardware will necessitate what software you purchase. Plan to have your low voltage wiring run a few months before construction is complete. Your contractor will run conduit within the floor and ceilings to allow low-voltage wiring pulls later in the construction process. Consult with your contractor on the best time to bring in a networking specialist. They will have to revisit your site after all the wiring is installed to setup your computer hardware, software and test its operations. The dry-run with friends and family will be another opportunity to iron out kinks in the software. Plan to have the software's representative onsite during this time to help with any problems in real-time.

You're on your way to a successful practice. Lean on your team, they are there to support you and take as much off your plate as possible.

- Peter Hays, Practice Real Estate Group

Chapter 4

Building A Strong Financial Foundation for a Successful Dental Practice

By Erick Cutler, CPA

As one of the leaders of our firm's health care practice, I'm approached by a great number of dentists for advice on setting up a new practice. There are so many things to discuss on this topic, including many areas the dentist may not have any knowledge of. This is why I appreciate the value of this book. It brings to light some of the essential areas for soon-to-be new practice owners. It begins to show the importance of building a solid team of professionals around the practice and the dentist not the least of which is the certified public accountant (CPA)/ financial advisor. The CPA relationship is one that should begin early while the new dental practice is still in the "thought process" and should continue well after the reins of the practice have been handed over to someone else. As a trusted advisor, a CPA who is familiar with the intricacies of running a dental practice like a business can become one of the dentist's closest confidants.

When engaged to consult with a dentist on opening a new practice, I like to begin by gaining a better understanding of the dentist. Asking questions and engaging in discussions around their specific area of practice, their length of time in practice, their experiences as a practitioner, what their expectations are with regard to practice ownership, and their level of nervousness or excitement around starting a new practice give profound insight into the who the dentist is.

However, keeping in mind why the dentist has come to me, I find it very important to ask questions about where he or she is in the process of this new venture. Do you know where you would like to locate your office? Have you spoken to a real estate professional that can not only help locate and secure space but can also provide demographic studies about the areas of interest to ensure it will support the type of practice the dentist wants to establish? Have you spoken to any lenders about the lending process, what that entails, and what information will be needed which could include pro forma financial statements, budgets, and forecasts? Have you spoken to any dental office designers or equipment representatives who will work very closely together during the construction process and to some extent for a short time after construction? Have you begun thinking about how you are going to get the word out to the public that you are open? How you are going to employ and train the new staff to properly handle the new patients from the first phone call to the first check in to the first time in the chair? All of this simply gives me more insight and understanding before I move to the final question that will occupy the remainder of the conversation: Have you put any thought into the financial structure of the practice and the financial reporting aspect of managing the practice as a business? What we are really talking about here is entity formation/selection and the importance of financial statement reporting.

When we talk about entity formation, we are talking about the incorporation of practice within the state where the practice is going to conduct business. For legal and financial reasons, this is something that should be done early on in the new practice startup life-cycle. The practice entity will the one "signing" the lease, potentially securing the practice loan, buying the equipment, and hiring the people that take care of the patients. Most dentists elect to form a professional limited liability company (PLLC), if it is available in their state, to be the practice's legal structure. This structure provides asset protection and flexibility for the owners of the practice but it does not determine how the practice will be treated for federal income tax purposes. To do that, the dentist, or more accurately the practice, must make one more election but this time with the Internal Revenue Service (IRS). It will elect to be treated as either a disregarded entity (a.k.a. sole proprietorship), C corporation, S corporation, or partnership.

- Disregarded entity does not file its own federal income tax return but reports everything on its owner's personal tax return by way of a Schedule C; income tax as well as self-employment tax is paid on any profit that the practice generates.

- C corp files its own income tax return, pays its own income taxes, and is a completely separate entity from the owners; the downside is double taxation (corporation and its owners pay income tax).

- S corp files its own income tax return but pays no federal income taxes; it is a pass-through entity which means the practice's profits or losses are "passed" through to shareholders/owners for reporting on their own personal tax returns. Shareholders can deduct losses only to the extent of their adjusted tax basis in the S corporation stock plus their adjusted tax basis in loans made directly to the S corporation by the shareholder. More times than not, single owner practices choose this election for its tax efficiency.

- Partnership is suggested for practices with multiple dentist owners and is also a pass-through entity with some of the same attributes as an S corporation but for the purposes of this discussion, we will not dive into those differences.

The decision to form a PLLC as the practice's legal structure is in most regards an easy one. However, the decision on what to elect for federal income tax purposes is not always so easy. Many factors such as the structure of the practice loan and the dentist's overall tax picture could influence which federal election is initially chosen. The good news is that elections can be changed but this does not alleviate the need to seek good counsel from your CPA from the outset. Elections can be changed but sometimes change is costly.

When it comes to managing the financial side of the practice or better still the business, there are few tools that are as good at showing the dentist where the practice has been, where it is, and where it is going rather than looking at the financial statements. The importance of the financial statements cannot be overstated. As mentioned earlier, pro forma financials or financials that model the expected results of a proposed transaction (starting a dental practice) may be required during the lending process. These very pro forma financials can become the backbone of the new practice's budget and cash flow models for helping the dentist make sure the new practice is performing as expected during those critical early months of operation. So, what exactly are financial statements, what do they tell us, and why are they important?

Financial statements are written records that convey the business activities and the financial performance of the practice and provide a snapshot of the practice's financial health, giving insight into its performance, operations, and cash flow. Financial statements are essential since they provide information about a practice's revenue, expenses, profitability, assets, and debt. They consist of three main components: balance sheet, income statement, and cash flow statement.

- **The Balance Sheet (a.k.a. Statement of Assets, Liabilities, and Capital)** is a snapshot in time. You could even look at it as the accounting version of a dental impression -- it tells you where things are at the moment it was prepared. It includes three main sections, the first of which is "assets." This section reports what the practice owns and is ideally ranked by how quickly those items can be converted into cash. The second section includes "liabilities," which is what the practice owes (to vendors, banks, etc.). These are also ideally ranked according to the due date. The third section is the "equity" or "capital" section. This section represents the residual value of the practice after all liabilities have been paid off. In other words, the practice's net worth.

- **The Income Statement (a.k.a. Profit and Loss Statement)** reports the profitability of the practice over a given period of time (usually the practice's fiscal year) by showing the total revenues and expenses for that time period. It is also a way to analyze how efficiently the practice is able to convert expenses into revenue. It's the financial statement that proves out the theory "you have to spend money to make money."

- **The Cash Flow Statement** reports the amount of cash flowing into and out of the practice. It measures how well the practice manages its cash position, meaning how well the practice generates cash to pay its debts and fund its operating expenses. This statement proves out the other popular theory "cash is king."

As a CPA and dental practice advisor, I understand that the dentist is first and foremost a doctor and a clinician so there is no need for the dentist to feel like they have to fully understand every line item on the financial statements. However, it is important to have a marginal level of comfort in reading these statements as they provide the base information for determining some of the most important key performance indicators (KPI) of the practice.

As you make examining your practice financials a habit, you will begin to get a good feel for how the practice is performing. You may even begin to see trends developing that will compel you to review them closer to uncover the "why" behind what you are seeing. Over time, certain KPIs will become more important to you than others; but to get you started, here are some of the most important for a new practice to keep an eye on. You'll be able to expand from here once you get comfortable pulling information from your statements and diving deeper into the meaning behind the numbers.

- **Budget vs. Actual:** Not so much a KPI as it is simply a great measurement tool to track how the practice is doing against the expectations set for it. Depending on the accounting software you use (i.e., QuickBooks) budgets can be entered into the software so that budget vs. actual reports can be run as part of your financial statement review process.

- **Profitability:** As elementary as it sounds, simply reviewing the profit and loss statement regularly will keep you aware of the profitability of the practice as a whole. As the practice matures, you can use the financial statements along with information from the practice management software to review profitability by procedure or provider.

- **Accounts Receivable:** This particular indicator found both on the balance sheet and in reports from the practice management software keeps track of the health of the collection process. A trend to be watchful of is a consistent increase month-to-month in the accounts receivable balance. This may not be a bad thing early on in the life of the practice as each month more patients are added than the previous month but keep an eye on it all the same.

- **Overhead:** Basically, what it costs to operate the practice. This is not the most technically correct definition of this indicator but it gets to the root of what you need to understand. Some specific overhead expenses to review regularly:

  ○ **Payroll:** Staffing and how much you are paying your staff. This delves into questions about compensation, production levels, hours, and overall staffing needs (under- or over-staffed). A good goal for staffing is around 25% of net production. If you feel the need to make adjustments, keep in mind that changes in this area impact the very culture of your practice.

  ○ **Lab fees:** This cost can vary greatly depending on your patient and service mix, but a good general goal is 6% of net production. You can adjust that number upward if you do a lot of work with crowns and other highly customized services.

  ○ **Dental Supplies:** The income statement should have this outlined clearly so that you're able to quickly assess how much you're spending, as well as how those expenditures fluctuate across the years. You should keep a guideline percentage (5% of net production is recommended) to use as a check against supply prices creeping up in comparison to what you're actually bringing in.

- **Marketing or Advertising:** Advertising generally shouldn't be included in your overhead. Unless you're just looking to maintain your current practice performance, you should be viewing advertising as an investment. You can consider spending as much as 10% in revenue on this area. Just make sure you're getting your money's worth by tracking effectiveness.

Although this last section was about financial statements and KPIs related to the financial statements, there are some other KPIs that I would be remiss if I didn't mention them and their importance to successful practice management. All of these can easily be pulled from the practice management software.

- Total Production
- Total Collection – a compliment to the review of the accounts receivables
- New Patient Referrals
- New Patient Conversions
- New Patient Count vs. Active Patient Count
- Hygiene Recall Appointments
- Treatment Acceptance

I am excited to be a part of this book. As I mentioned earlier, I appreciate the value this book brings to dentists who are ready to strike out on their own and start a new dental practice by bringing together a team of professionals well versed in the area of dental practice startup. Furthermore, having that trusted advisor who is familiar with the intricacies of running a dental practice as a business will become one of the dentist's most important resources. The ability to provide guidance throughout the life of the practice will be invaluable whether it is applied to reviewing and interpreting the vast amount of critical information reported on the financial statements of the practice or diving into the KPIs that tell the story of the practice. This process should be an exciting and enjoyable venture but is not one to go into alone. Rely on the experience of your professionals to help make sure the practice begins with a head start.

Eric Cutler is a Tax Partner at EisnerAmper LLC.

TOOTH FAIRY DENTAL PLLC
Profit & Loss
January through December 2020 and 2019

	Jan - Dec 2020	Jan - Dec 2019	$ Change
Ordinary Income/Expense			
Income			
Revenue			
Tooth Fairy	$ 188,845	$ 236,985	$ (48,140)
Deposit	964,440	315,825	648,615
Total Revenue	1,153,285	552,810	600,475
Sales Return/Refunds	(121)	-	(121)
Total Income	1,153,164	552,810	600,354
Cost of Goods Sold			
Cost of sales			
Dental Supplies	53,740	15,089	38,651
Lab Expense	40,318	7,811	32,507
Cost of Sales	94,058	22,900	71,158
Total Cost of Goods Sold	94,058	22,900	71,158
Gross Profit	1,059,106	529,910	529,196
Expense			
Advertising	13,750	470	13,280
Auto Expenses	678	4,807	(4,129)
Auto Lease	8,026	5,096	2,930
Parking and Tolls	50	1,143	(1,093)
Bank Charges	12,750	4,284	8,466
Business Licenses & Permits	1,664	2,466	(802)
Computer and Internet Expenses	1,513	829	684
Continuing Education	275	1,464	(1,189)
Contract Labor	1,404	19,904	(18,500)
Credit Card Fees	525	525	-
Donations	500	685	(185)
Dues & Subscriptions	95	125	(30)
Gifts	65	65	-
Insurance - Health	8,934	9,373	(439)
Insurance - Others	7,340	7,902	(562)
Janitorial & Cleaning	2,459	551	1,908
Legal & Accounting Fees	5,946	4,700	1,246
Meal & Entertainment	4,540	12,130	(7,590)
Office Expenses	4,777	11,178	(6,401)
Payroll Expenses	401	115	286
Payroll Taxes	21,099	12,208	8,891
Postage	1,070	1,171	(101)
Rent Expense	78,795	44,397	34,398
Repairs & Maintenance	3,842	2,033	1,809
Salaries and Wages	184,501	64,020	120,481
Security Expenses	458	985	(527)
Small Dental Equipment	608	-	608
Taxes - Others	286	287	(1)
Telephone	1,425	2,559	(1,134)
Travel	525	14,521	(13,996)
Utilities	7,750	2,992	4,758
Uniforms	245	-	245
Total Expense	376,296	232,985	143,311
Net Ordinary Income	682,810	296,925	385,885
Other Income/Expense			
Other Income			
Interest Income	7	-	7
Total Other Income	7	-	7
Other Expense			
Interest Expense	27,145	11,330	15,815
Amortization	22,400	11,200	11,200
Depreciation	5,762	191,731	(185,969)
Officer Salary	66,000	72,000	(6,000)
Total Other Expense	121,307	286,261	(164,954)
Net Other Expense	(121,300)	(286,261)	164,961
Net Income	561,510	10,664	550,846

Example Income Statement

Chapter 5
Office Design and Construction

by William Cruz

This chapter, will focus on the process of designing and constructing a new dental office. The goal is to provide a basic understanding of the processes that take place between selecting your office location and a move-in day. A chronological approach will be laid out, starting directly after you have met with your real estate broker.

The design team gets involved after you have found a possible location. This can be either a piece of land, known as a ground-up building, or a retail center; called a finish out. We'll go into further detail on what each of these types of projects entail in the rest of this chapter.

Regardless of the type of a project and once your design team is engaged, the first step is completing a "Wish List" for the project. The Wish List is a short questionnaire that identifies the doctor's vision for the practice, including and not limited to the number of operatories, open bay chairs, offices, and staff meeting areas. This questionnaire is an invaluable and will serve as a starting point for our design team.

1. Ground up buildings

Ground ups are when the dentist buys a piece of land and has a team design their practice from scratch, literally, from the ground up! On these projects, the design team begins by examining a survey of the land and determining the setbacks, egress, parking lot restrictions, etc.

Once an overall parameter for the footprint of the building has been determined, the team examines the Wish List and starts the work on the preliminary design. Ground up buildings are large projects that entail the assistance of engineers, site architects and a whole team of people to take the project off the ground. They take 4 to 5 times longer than a finish out space, and cost significantly more.

The cost for ground up buildings costing anywhere between 200-350 dollars per square ft. The price is determined by how much work the site needs, whether the city lines (water, sewer, and electricity) are nearby or need to be brought in from a further distance.

As it is probably clear by now, ground up buildings are more complex projects that entail a lot of time, money and expertise. In my opinion, these projects should be undertaken by those who already have a thriving practice and who would like to now own their building.

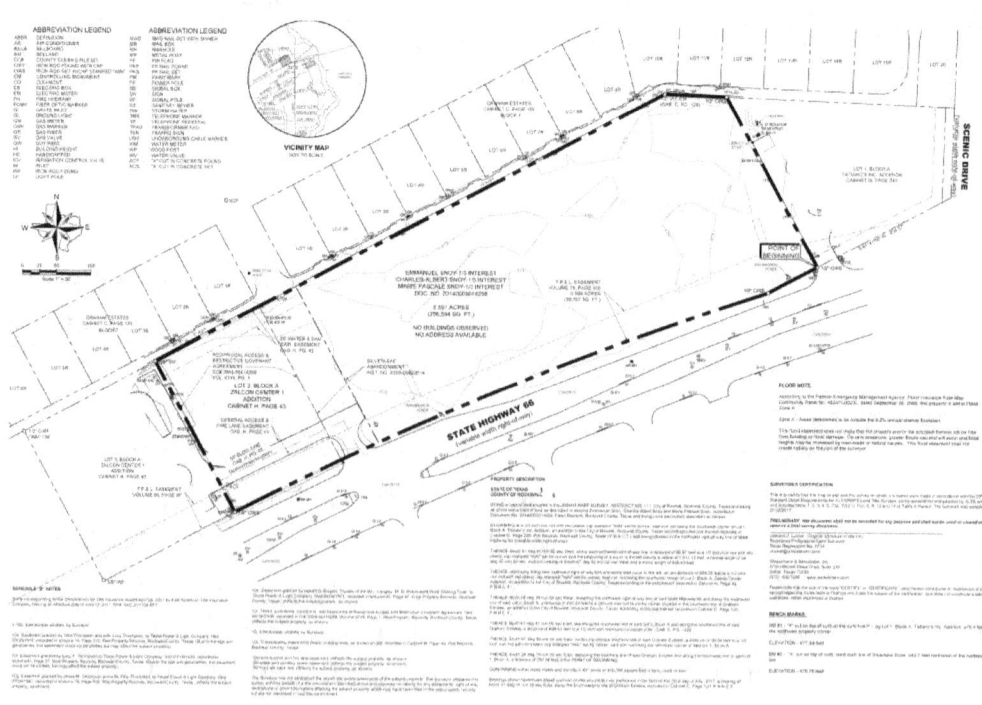

2. Finish out spaces

If this is going to be your first start up, a finish out project is the best option. They are a lot more common and offer a straightforward process. You and your broker will find a suite at a location you like, usually in a retail center, and provide a floor plan of the shell of the building — see the picture below as an example. The brokers we associate with conduct several demographic studies of the region in order to determine a suitable location for our client. Once the location is selected, you will meet with our team. Together we go over the design process, complete the Wish List and begin the work on the preliminary design of the dental office.

We are often asked, "How large of a space do I need?" This isn't a cut and dry question, as there are several factors to consider: type of practice (general practitioner, pediatric dentist, oral surgeon, etc.), size of the operatories, size of the waiting room, or whether or not the doctor wants a private restroom inside their private office, for instance. Generally, our designs take about 350-400 sq ft per operatory. So, for example, a building that's 3000 sq ft will accommodate around 7-8 OPs.

Finish out spaces have a smaller range of cost per square ft; they cost anywhere between 90-120 dollars per square ft. In addition, the doctors get a TI allowance (tenants improvements) from the landlord to help with that cost. The allowances in urban areas range from 25-40 dollars per square ft, depending on how desirable and how much exposure a space has.

Designing the office is a collaborative process. You explain your vision for the practice, and the design team translates that into a cohesive design that takes this into consideration, along with the overall flow of the office, building standards, local buildings codes, and both federal and state accessibility codes.

In order to best capture your vision for the practice, it is important to explore what the finished project will look like before construction even takes place. To do this, you should be provided with 3D renditions and virtual tours of your office. We have found that this is the best tool for ensuring that everyone is happy with the finished project before the work begins and avoids costly last-minute changes.

The 3D renderings and virtual tours are a tool for evaluating the flow of the office and scale of the rooms. Selection of finishes and materials does not happen at allowances in urban areas range from 25-40 dollars per square ft, depending on how desirable and how much exposure a space has.

The typical submittals of a preliminary design constitute 12-15 renderings of the practice, a virtual tour of the space and the floor plan. See below for some examples.

Once a preliminary design is submitted, you'll go over it and see what you do and do not like. Once we get a list of items that need to be addressed our team starts on the design revisions. On each revision, we submit the same folder with renderings and virtual tours of the space; as always, the goal is to explore any shortcomings of the floor plan during the design stage. The preliminary design stage usually takes a couple of weeks — about 2 days for each revision — and communication between the doctor and the design team is key to ensure a

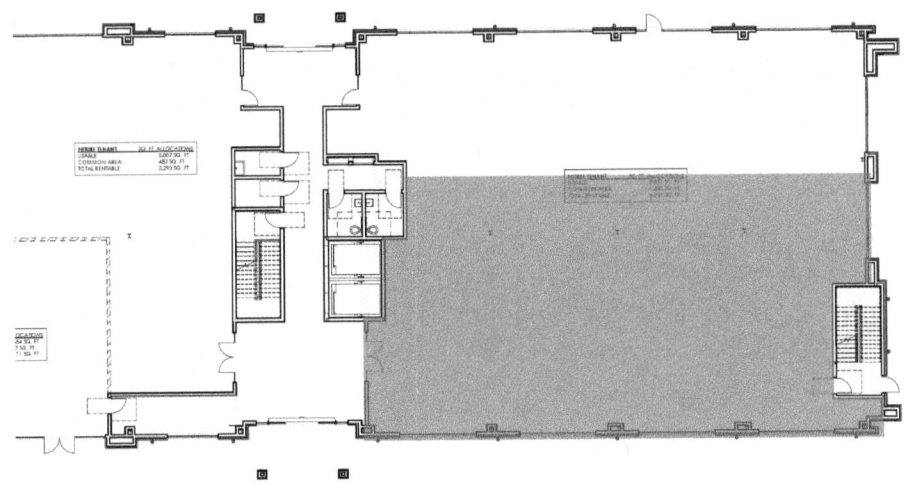

Landlord provided file

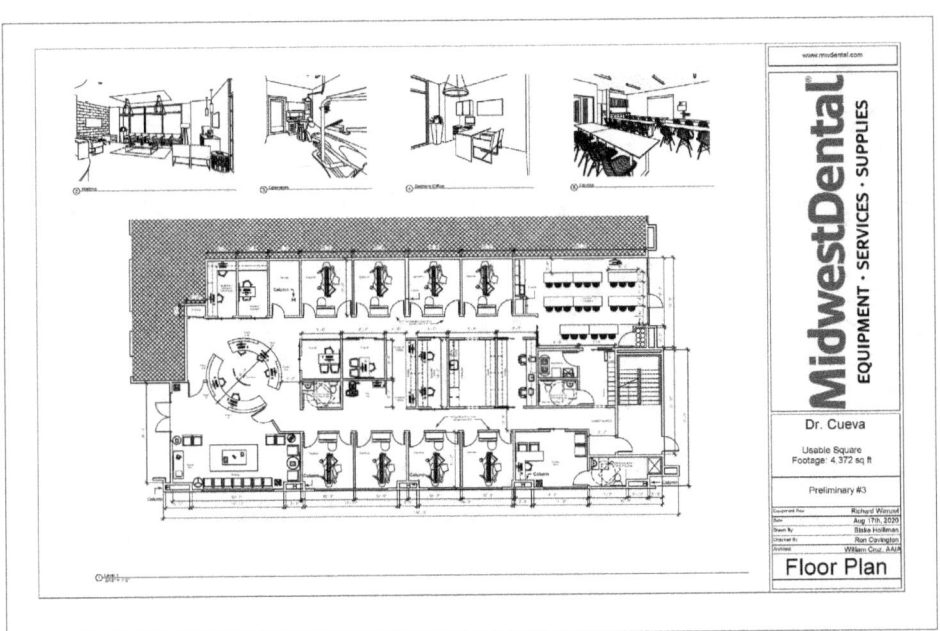

For more examples of office layouts visit;
https://the2hourdentalstartup.com/portfolio/

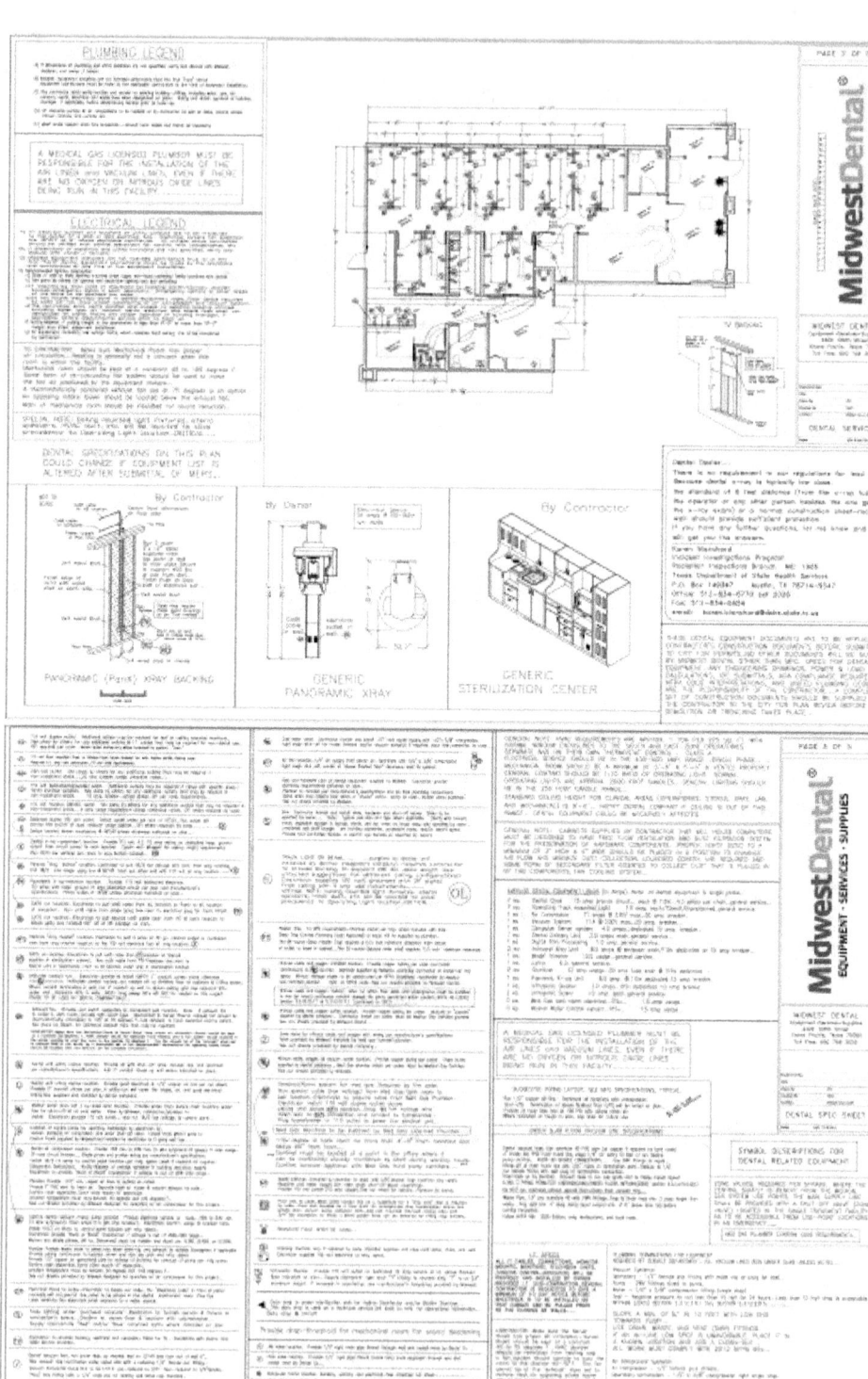

successful design. At the end of this stage, both the designer and the doctor should understand the different possibilities of the space and have a firm idea of what the space will look like once built. This is when we move to the Dental MEPs stage of the process.

3. Dental MEPs stage

During the Dental MEPs stage, the design team incorporates all the necessary information regarding the dental equipment into the design. In other words, we get a list of the dental equipment you have decided to use in your new practice, and everything that's needed to make said equipment run properly.

The Dental MEPs show the contractor where the air (drive gas), vacuum, and electrical lines need to be located. In addition, they show details on how they need to be run, the size of the lines and the termination locations. They will also show backing, venting and drainage information. In short, they give the contractors the information they need to properly bid for the projects and avoid any surprises during construction, such as change orders.

It is important to know that the Dental MEPs are not construction or permit drawings; those will be done by the contractors later on in the process.

Regarding finishes, the contractor sets up a system of allowances for you. The contractor provides several options for materials that are within the allowance from which to make your selection - and upgrades are always permissible at an additional cost.

With the Dental MEPs in hand, you are now ready to get bids from contractors. The Dental MEPs are sent to the con-

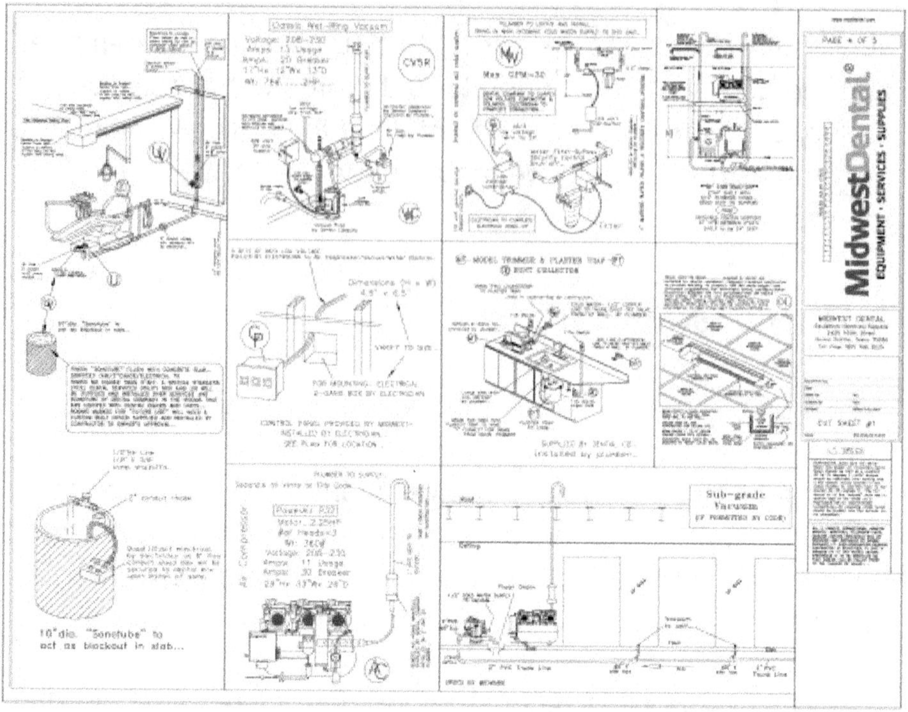

Odntd Wet-Ring Vacuum

CV5R

MW

B- MODEL TRIMMER & PLASTER TRAP
DIRT COLLECTOR

MidwestDental®
EQUIPMENT · SERVICES · SUPPLIES

MIDWEST DENTAL

CUT SHEET #1

Air Compressor

Sub-grade
Vacuum
(IF PERMITTED BY CODE)

10" dia. "Sonotube" to
act as blockout in slab...

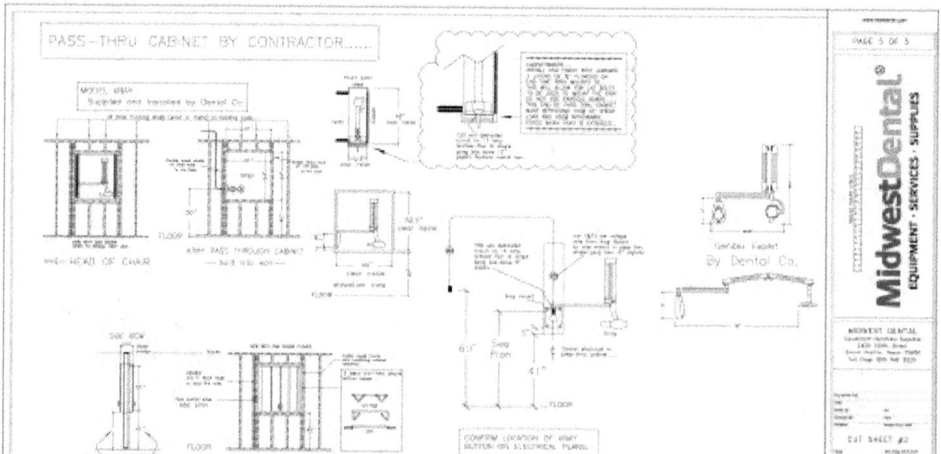

PASS-THRU CABINET BY CONTRACTOR.....

MODEL XXXX
Supplied and Installed by Dental Co.

HEAD OF CHAIR

X-RAY PASS THROUGH CABINET

SIDE VIEW

FOOT OF CHAIR

Cabinet Light
By Dental Co.

CONFIRM LOCATION OF X-RAY
SECTION ON ELECTRICAL PLANS

MidwestDental®
EQUIPMENT · SERVICES · SUPPLIES

MIDWEST DENTAL

CUT SHEET #2

tractors in both PDF and CAD formats. The contractors go over the detailed drawings, get quotes from their sub-contractors, and material costs from their vendors prior to submitting their bid for the project. This process typically takes around 2 weeks.

One main advantage of getting bids straight from contractors is that it gives you the ability to value-engineer a project. Because the finishes have not been selected yet, the contractors are able to give you options from their preferred vendors in order to maximize your budget. After meeting the contractors and getting their bids, you can

review the bids and decide which contractor you would prefer to work with. This takes us to the next phase of our process.

4. Construction drawings & permits

Most dental contractors have an in-house drafting team who prepare the permit drawings. They take the Dental MEPs, renderings, and notes from their meetings with the clients, and start on the construction/permit drawings. This set of drawings is typically around 15 pages long (triple that amount for a ground up building) and consist of detailed drawings from the electrician, plumbers, HVAC, etc. Depending on the square footage and municipality, this set of drawings might then need to be sealed by an Engineer/Architect. This stage of the process typically takes around 2 weeks and, in most cases, does not accrue any additional costs as most dental contractors offer it as part of their package.

Once the construction drawings are finalized, they are submitted for permits. Smaller cities tend to have a faster review process, maybe 4 weeks or so, while larger municipalities (Houston, for example) can take as long as 9-10 weeks to finalize their permitting process. This stage of the process is generally handled by the contractors and requires very little input from the doctor — which is not to say that the doctor is idle! While this takes place, the doctor typically meets with the contractors to select finishes (colors & materials) for the project.

5. Site-checks & Equipment Installation

During construction, a number of site checks need to be performed to ensure that our dental MEPs are being followed (not all equipment companies offer this service). Often, you'll be able to meet us on one of these site checks so we can answer whatever questions you might have. After construction is complete, our lead technician does a pre-installation check to make sure that everything is ready for the installation of the dental equipment. Installation then begins, which in most cases takes between 3 to 4 days.

Once the dental equipment is installed, the design team, equipment representative, and install crew takes a step back and your account supply representative will become your trusted advisor throughout your career.

Chapter 6

Equipment Selection - Choosing the Right Equipment

by Eric Swarvar

Next to construction, dental equipment is the largest investment in the start-up process. The total cost of ownership(TCO) needs to be considered when making a purchasing decision. TCO = original purchase price + cost of operating and maintenance. It also assesses the value of the equipment over the lifespan of ownership. I would like to make it very clear I have evaluated numerous practices that the owner in 30+ years never reinvested in their equipment. Yes, patients know that the chair is 30 years old and it looks old. The life expectancy of equipment under general conditions is approximated at:

Operatory equipment: 10-15 years
Mechanical closet: 12-15 years
Sterilizer: 10,000 cycles
Handpieces: 5-7 years
Ultrasonic Scaler: 7-10 years
ProphyJet: 5 years
Digital sensor: 5-7 years
Computers: update every 5 years

Proper maintenance and frequency of use should also be considered when determining equipment life expectancy.

Maintenance Closet

The maintenance closet of a dental office is generally misunderstood. There are two pieces of equipment inside the closet that powers the operator equipment: the dental air compressor and the dental vacuum. An easy phrase to remember the purpose of each piece of equipment is, "Vacuums suck and compressors blow."

All dental compressors and vacuums are measured in users and not operatories. When a compressor is rated at 2-3 users, this is defined as 2-3 operators putting a demand on the compressor simultaneously. An example of this would be a 5 operatory practice with one doctor and two dental hygienists. This would require a minimum of a 3 operator unit. It is a good idea to plan for the future. If you are a solo practitioner looking to expand, having a larger vacuum and compressor is better. Other considerations should be location of compressor and vacuum. The further the units from the clinic setting the harder the units will work. Also, putting a vacuum upstairs will diminish the strength of the unit.

The Dental Air Compressor: Only an oil free dental air compressor should be used for drive air inside a dental practice. Dental compressors are configured specifically to filter out dust and bacteria contaminants and provide dry fresh air for dental surgical use. Do not use a construction compressor, as you will set yourself up for failure and disappointment. Construction compressors do not have the necessary components to create dental drive air.

Dental vacuums: Dry vacuums and wet ring vacuums are the two types of vacuums we will discuss. (An air compressor can also be used to create a vacuum, however is only used in oral surgery. For the purpose of this book we will focus on the two types of dental vacuums) A wet ring vacuum uses water to create vacuum pressure, using an average of over 320 gallons a day. A dry vacuum uses rotary fins to create a suction with no water. More expensive up front, the dry vacuum can have less TCO than a wet ring vacuum, especially if you are paying for your own water. An additional item included in your mechanical closet is a water-shut-off-solenoid which also includes a water-filter-by-pass system. This mechanism filters out the macro particles in your system and allows you to shut off the water to the building with the push of a button. This is important to prevent any potential flooding.

Connected to the vacuum is an amalgam separator. On July 14, 2020, the EPA mandated 40 CFR Part 441 requiring most dental offices to have an amalgam separator. The state and local water municipalities are charged with enforcement of this regulation. Please note even if you do not place amalgam you must have a separator, with the exception of these specialists:

- Oral pathology
- Oral and maxillofacial radiology
- Oral and maxillofacial surgery
- Orthodontics
- Periodontics
- Prosthodontics
- Mobile dental clinics
- Facilities that discharge in to septic systems.

Operatory Equipment

Dental chairs are the focus of every operatory and evaluated on comfort and esthetic. There are two types of lifting mechanisms for dental chairs: hydraulic cantilever and electromechanical cantilever. Most chairs use a hydraulic cantilever system, which gives a more consistent source of power for lifting the patient. There are also several types of upholstery available on the market. One is standard vinyl upholstery which is limited in colors. The other is upgraded upholstery (sold under various brands) which generally provides an endless color selection. Now that you have your color and quality selection of upholstery, style options are next, which is asepsis (vacuum sealed no stitching) or plush (seamed stitched upholstery). Additional choices can include size of backing on the dental chair, arm slings, and color of base.

Some important notes are most chairs have upholstery kits available that replace not only the upholstery, but also the cushion. Over time, replacing the upholstery with an upholstery kit can freshen up the look in your operatory. You should also clean your dental upholstery several times a month to prevent any chemical build up from your disinfectant, ensuring the longterm care and look of your upholstery.

There are several styles of delivery and for the purpose of this book they will be described based on their position in the operatory.

• 12 o'clock position is the most common style of delivery. This includes the operators delivery equipment positioned behind the operator. This provides a less intimidated look for nervous patients and allows access for all surgical delivery mounted to a cabinet, counter, cart, or pedestal.

• Over the patient delivery is the second most popular style of delivery. This is an operator delivery mounted to the chair. There are two styles of this type of delivery: swing mount delivery and fixed. Swing mount delivery swings from a pivot point at the toe of the chair. This is useful to provided delivery for left and right handed operators. Fixed mounted on the chair is a unit mounted to a post. A single side of the chair is chosen for this mounting location, providing limited delivery for either a left or right handed dentist, but not both. Over the patient delivery is seen as an appropriate ergonomic solution in dentistry.

• Side delivery is another option of delivery, mounted to a side wall. The location is selected based on the handedness of the operator. If the operator is left handed the delivery will be mounted on the left wall or the 3 o'clock position. If they are right handed the delivery will be mounted on the right wall or the 6 o'clock position. This is truly an operators preference with no profound benefit to build an office based on this style of delivery.

Types of delivery

• Doctors delivery - Most modern dental delivery units are automatic units, utilizing pneumatic switches that activate a particular handpiece location when that device is removed from it's holder. Another option is an analog system, utilizing a selector switch forcing the practitioner to hit a switch every time they want to use that particular handpiece. Doctor delivery units include an air-water syringe and has several positions for handpieces (generally 3) one with fiber optics for illumination of light from a dental handpiece, and two other handpiece tubings, one for low-speed handpieces and a second position for either surgical or back-up high-speed. Other items to consider on the doctors delivery is integration of technology to include; electric handpiece with or without endo-capability, curing light, surgical piezo, hygiene ultrasonic scaler, and restorative material handpiece. Remember the more factory integration options, the harder it will be to uninstall and send the item in for service. A quality delivery unit should include a water selector switch that allows the practitioner to eliminate the water, water adjustment valves allowing the individual to increase or decrease the amount of water coming out the handpiece, chip air adjustment, and a purge valve to remove the left over water from the lines at the end of the day. Doctors delivery units do NOT include assistant's package.

- Hygiene delivery is a delivery unit that is a little more stripped down with an air-water syringe and two 4 hole handpiece tubings with no illumination. The unit also includes an evacuation system with one saliva-ejector valve, one high-volume-evacuation valve, and a collection canister that holds a solids trap. Factory integration of an ultrasonic scaler is possible with this style of delivery. This unit should have a master switch to turn it on, a water selector valve, and a purge switch to remove any leftover water in the lines at the end of the day.
- Assistant's package includes an air-water syringe with a saliva-ejector valve, 1-2 high volume evacuation valves, and a collection canister that houses a vacuum trap to catch any large particles. Typically these items are mounted on some type of arm. The location of this package is determined on the location of the doctors delivery and ability to run the evacuation lines during the construction phase. The 12 o'clock position is generally the most common location. Some assistant packages utilize an integrated work surface,

providing the dental assistant with a more universal work surface.
  • Bonus info: if you want the driest air out of your air water syringe have a single button syringe included in your delivery unit, only connect an air line to this syringe.

All delivery systems should utilize a self-contained bottle system as the water source to the delivery unit. This allows the clinician to control the quality of water entering the delivery system, treat the dental water lines, and operate if there is a boil water notice. Various sizes and numerous bottles are available.

Operatory Lighting

Because the patient does not have a light on the dorsal of their tongue, lighting is always important in the clinical setting. There are 4 primary sources of lighting in the operatory. Ambient light is installed during the construction process which will provide general light in the room but not enough to do a class II restoration. Color temperature is measured by Kelvin degrees. Natural sunlight measures in the range of 5,500°K. You don't want your employees wearing sunglasses inside all day so shoot for somewhere in the 4,500°K range. The color rendering index (CRI) is measured by percentages and the sun is the standard at 100%. The lower the percentage, the more yellow the light. Think 1970's death cubicle corporate America. Ideally you should shoot for a CRI of 100%.

The primary light source to illuminate the oral cavity is the dental operatory light.
• Track style is the most common as it has more flexibility. The light is mounted on a track and can be slid to the toe of the chair to be out of the way when the patient enters or exits the chair.
• A ceiling mounted light is a light fixed to the ceiling that can only swing out of the way.

- A pole mounted light is mounted to the chair and is the least expensive option. Even the slightest movement in the chair can cause the light to shake and can distract the focus of the clinician while working.
- A wall mounted light can also be used but is the least desirable as a bar running parallel holds the light head in place. This takes up too much space and can be a limiter for the assistant. Most modern operatory lights use a light emitting diode that have multiple intensities and touch switches to activate. A no cure setting is considered a luxury, but is a very nice addition for any dentist.

Dental handpiece illumination should be standard when selecting high-speed handpieces. This additional illumination will reduce any shadowing in the oral cavity.

Another light source option is the headlight mounted to loupes or a headband. In recent times, some dentist have opted to not install an operatory light and only use their optic mounted light as their main source. This can pose a problem for the assistant as they will also need to have a headlight.

Nitrous Delivery

There are two styles of nitrous delivery, plumbed nitrous and cart style. Plumbed style has nitrous and oxygen plumbed through the entire clinic setting. Not all chairs need to be plumbed but in most cases the cost is negligible. A manifold, flowmeter, alarm panel, zone valve, cylinder regulator for each tank, and a cylinder restrain system is all needed for plumbed nitrous. A plumbed system uses G&H tanks. Plumbed should only be considered when extensive construction is involved in the entirety of the project. If nitrous is used on the majority of the patients (pediatric office) plumbed nitrous is the clear choice.

Cart style is a self-contained cart that uses multiple E-style tanks. E-style tanks generally are 4X more expensive to fill than

G&H tanks. A cart needs to be hooked up to a vacuum valve for proper scavenging. Cart style is perfect for the practice that wants access to nitrous but does not use it frequently.

Dental Handpieces

The number of handpieces a practitioner should start with is a minimum of 4:
- One in use
- One in the sterilizer
- One sterile for the next patient
- One sterile for back-up.

This philosophy should be used for high and low speed handpieces, as the CDC has mandated each device to include hygiene handpieces be sterilized after each patient.

Multiple semi-critical dental devices that touch mucous membranes are attached to the air or waterlines of the dental unit. Among these devices are high- and low-speed handpieces, prophylaxis angles, ultrasonic and sonic scaling tips, air abrasion devices, and air and water syringe tips.

There are two types of high and low-speed handpieces: electric and air driven.

Air driven handpieces have existed since the 1950's, utilizing air flowing over a finned turbine to operate the dental bur. The feathering technique is taught because of this handpiece. When touched to the tooth after a few seconds the pressure against the tooth slows the turbine down, forcing the practitioner to remove from the tooth to allow the turbine to speed up again. Most of these handpieces can hit above 300,000 RPM but typically operate below that. Air driven low speeds utilize a motor to drive the handpiece and not a turbine. A separate motor must me purchased to drive low speeds. Since that motor is attached to air and water it must be sterilized after each patient, requiring the practitioner to purchase multiple motors.

An electric motor is utilized to provide a constant RPM giving better cutting performance with an electric handpiece. Electric handpieces have the versatility to operate between 20 - 200,000 RPM. A practitioner does not have to utilize the feathering technique with this style of handpiece. The practitioners prep-style is more like a milling motion. Most companies that manufacture electric handpieces have endodontic settings that can utilize an endo-attachment. This feature eliminates the need for a separate motor for rotary-endo. Since the low speed attachments use the same electronic motor as the high speed, no separate motor needs to be purchased for low speed.

When adhering with the CDC standard of infection control, factoring in the cost of the appropriate amount of handpieces, electric handpieces are less expensive for a start-up than air-driven.

Intra-oral X-ray

There are essentially two types of intra-oral x-ray emitting devices:
• Wall mounted
• Portable

A wall mounted X-ray is mounted to a wall to stabilize the unit limiting it to one location. A pass-through cabinet can be utilized so the X-ray can be shared between operatories. The cabinet and bracing adds to the cost of the unit by about 25%.

Portable x-ray units are most associated with a battery operated handheld device. This gives the operator the flexibility for it to be used anywhere in the clinic. This unit carries its own host of problems like damage from dropping it, battery discharging, and generally offices under purchase the number of units. Intra-oral digital X-ray sensors are the standard in dentistry and have decreased the amount of time it takes to get diagnostic X-rays. The image quality is far superior to analog film and with modern software, multiple filters can make the diagnostic capability much easier. Displaying an X-ray image on a large monitor in the operatory is a vital tool to increase the acceptance ratio.

Panoramic/CBCT X-ray

Panoramic, pan/ceph, and CBCT are the 3 types of panoramic X-rays available on the market. The type of procedures performed inside the clinicians practice should determine what unit to choose.

A basic panoramic X-ray will provide the clinician with a window into the patients head, neck, and jaw. Some of these units have extra-oral bite-wing capabilities giving the practitioner a second option in capturing these shots on a difficult patient.

Pan/Ceph is designed for orthodontic use and gives extended diagnostics value for expanded insight.

Cone beam computed tomography CBCT is quickly becoming the standard of care in dentistry. CBCT creates a 3D image giving the clinician access to information that otherwise could only be obtained by a scalpel. Field of view, scan time, imaging software, and support are important features that need to be considered when making this decision. These units are regulated differently in each state and I advise to check with local and state codes when making a commitment to this technology.

Sterilization equipment

Once production is humming along, the sterilization area is the bottle neck of the clinical setting. An efficient area will include either an ultrasonic cleaner or an instrument washer as a device to clean any debris off the instruments. Once rinsed, the devices need to be maintained. Lubed hinges, surgical milk bath, and handpiece maintenance need to be considered. An automated handpiece maintenance station should be utilized to oil and purge all handpieces where it is required. This will protect the investment of handpieces and streamline the maintenance procedure. Afterwards, the devices are put into a sterilizer for processing. The automatic sterilizer utilizes steam technology to kill all organisms to prevent cross-contamination. There are multiple types of sterilizers from basic manual units to Class B sterilizers that vacuum out ambient air in the process. Chambered sterilizers provide more volume for instruments while cassette sterilizers tend to be quicker. A combination of both is an ideal for capacity.

Instrument cassettes provide a streamlined process to protect the investment of dental instruments and your team from any unwanted sticks. This process utilizes an optimal environment for transporting, cleaning, and sterilizing instruments.

For the purpose of this book we have only discussed the major clinical equipment. Below are some miscellaneous items not discussed.

- Lab Lathe with hoods
- Model trimmer
- Lab vent
- Lab handpiece
- AED
- Pulse Oximeter
- Blood Pressure device
- Laser

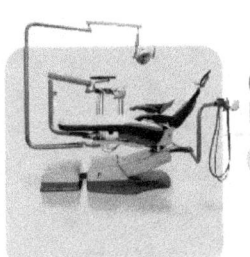

OPERATORY
EQUIPMENT

10-15 YEARS

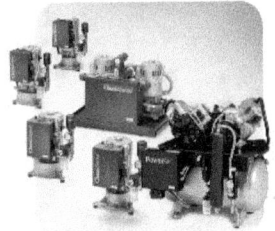

MECHANICAL
CLOSET

12-15 YEARS

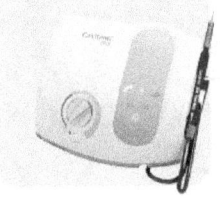

ULTRASONIC SCALER

7-10 YEARS

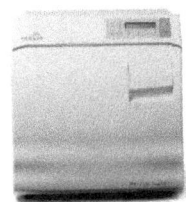

STERILIZER

10,000 CYCLES

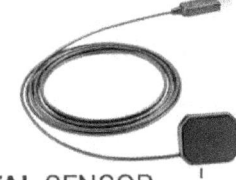

DIGITAL SENSOR

5-7 YEARS

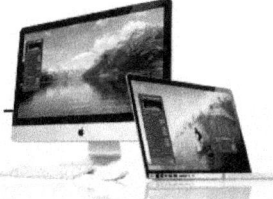

COMPUTERS

UPDATE EVERY
5-7 YEARS

HANDPIECES

5-7 YEARS

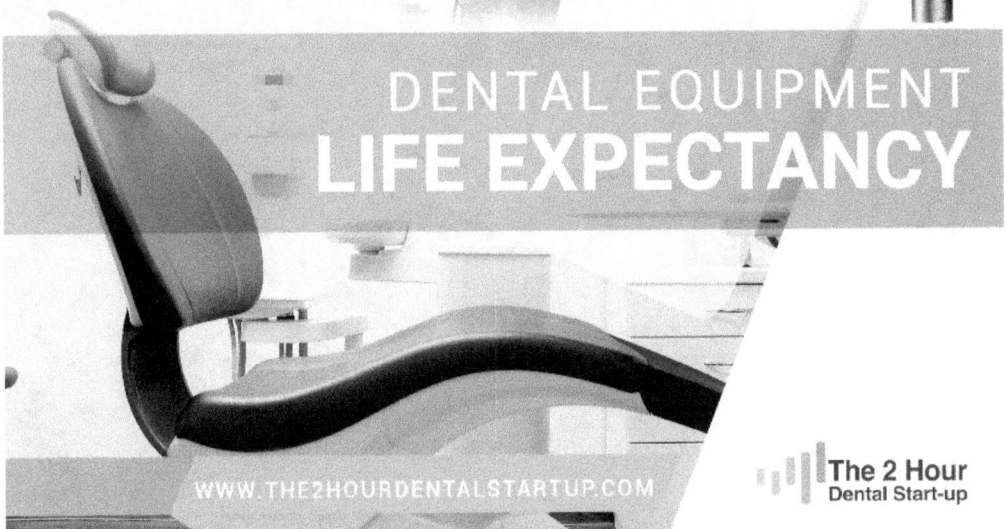

DENTAL EQUIPMENT
LIFE EXPECTANCY

WWW.THE2HOURDENTALSTARTUP.COM

The 2 Hour
Dental Start-up

- CAD/CAM

EQUIPMENT LIST

1 VACUUM **TYPE**
Wet Ring   DryVac

2 AIR **COMPRESSOR**
2-3 users   3-5 users   5-7 users   8-10 users

3 **DELIVERY**
Rear   Over the patient   Side Mount   Cart

4 OPERATORY **LIGHT**
Ceiling Mounted   Track Mounted
Side Mounted   Chair mounted   None

5 **NITROUS/MEDGAS**
Plumbed   Carts   NONE

6 EXTRAORAL **X-RAY**
Panoramic   Pan/Ceph   CBCT

7 INTRAORAL **X-RAY**
Size 1   Size2   Size1.5

8 **HANDPIECE**
Electric   Air Driven

9 STERILIZATION **ORGANIZATION CASSETTES**
Yes   No

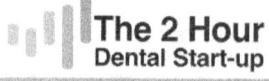
The 2 Hour
Dental Start-up

WWW.THE2HOURDENTALSTARTUP.COM

Chapter 7

Ground Marketing

by Michael Arias

I want you to envision your practice?

You are inside your practice and you are walking out of the front doors into the parking lot..,

You look to your left and you see a coffee shop, a grocery store, some small businesses.... And then you look to your right you see corporations... behind your practice are some apartments and homes... in front of your practice is another shopping strip where there are other small businesses and restaurants.... A couple blocks down there is a school, gym, day cares, senior homes and more locations.

You stand outside and you are thinking to yourself:

"I wonder how I can get those employees/ members/ residents/ customers to come to my practice"?

Well...that's where Ground Marketing comes in.

Ground Marketing is a sophisticated way of Guerrilla Marketing where you are getting the employee, residents, members, and customers to come to your practice with little to no cost.

You see the scenario above happened to me.

I was that person who walked out of the practice I worked in and wondered this. The doctor who I worked for did not have any money to put into marketing. I remember she literally said to me: "I can either hire an agency and fire you... or I can pay you your salary, and somehow you will bring me more new patients immediately".

That was it.

I was determined to find a way to get into these locations and bring in new patients immediately... and I did.

I created systems, scripts, tactics, and strategies that I am going to share with you here in this chapter.

These Ground Marketing strategies WILL bring you more new patients.

But first, I want to quickly break down what Ground Marketing is NOT!

Many of us (*especially back in the day*) would get some goodies, maybe cookies, or a gift basket and go to a small business... introduce ourselves... let them know *we are now accepting new patients*... drop off the gift baskets and then leave.

We would feel good about this because maybe the small business we left the gift basket too seemed positive... however days and weeks passed and you wouldn't hear from that business again.

That is NOT Ground Marketing. Although that may feel good and bring you hope... **hope doesn't pay the bills.** Butts in your chairs pay the bills!

Ground Marketing is a secure way for you to get some sort of exchange and contact information from the locations you visit. <u>I never want you to just drop stuff off and leave referral pads hoping people will call you.</u> You must always have the ball in your court.

I will teach you how to ALWAYS come out of these locations with names and numbers of people wanting to go to your practice.

Now that we got that out of the way let's start diving into it!

Ground Marketing is extremely useful for any practice, whether you are just starting out or you have been open for decades. It will create brand awareness, you will be seen more as an authority figure in your community, and of course you will bring in new patients.

There are 2 rules when Ground Marketing. This is something I burn into my students mind when they are out performing strategies.

Rule #1: Never Assume

Rule #2: Always Execute

Many times, and I speak from experience, we have paralysis by analysis and then we tend to tell ourselves something won't work without even trying it.

So don't assume... and try it. Execute.

Now since we are talking about start-ups I am going to focus on a couple key strategies that will work perfectly for you, especially as a start-up.

We will discuss three things:

1. Where To Start Ground Marketing
2. Ground Marketing to Apartments
3. How To Do a Grand Opening/ Open House During COVID-19

Let dive in.

WHERE TO START GROUND MARKETING

Now, this question comes to me probably a dozen times a week. We all want to start Ground Marketing but, where do you start?

Do you just start giving out fruit baskets to your neighbors? Do you hand out your pamphlets and business cards to the shopping strip across from you?!

I put it this way:

Let's say you are hungry and you go to the grocery store, with no grocery list, and no budget... what happens? Well, since you are hungry you probably tend to get the foods that look the most appealing but are they the healthiest options (probably not). Then you start to get random groceries even like, chips, some fruit, maybe some uncooked salmon, some deli meat, and bread (in case the salmon doesn't come out right you can make sandwiches, right)? Then you go to checkout and realize the total of the groceries is a lot more than you expected... but you pay anyways. You go home eat the bag of chips and some sandwiches and then your'e no longer hungry.

So, what groceries do you have for the rest of the week? Salmon, fruit, and bread. Now, you have realized you over spent on your grocery budget, didn't get food that made sense to your health goals, and you didn't get enough food for the week.

What should you have done? You should have created a grocery list BEFORE you started getting hungry, created a budget for the groceries, and gone out to get the groceries for the week.

Same thing... if you go blindly, thinking you are Ground Marketing to the right places and businesses, you start doing random things like "dropping off gift baskets" because you think this works here and there, ... then you'll just be spending time, money, and energy on things that won't produce real results or long term results (new patients in your practice).

So, in this section we will learn where to start with Ground Marketing.

I am going to teach you how to start with three basic steps... ready?

STEP ONE: *PLAN AHEAD.*

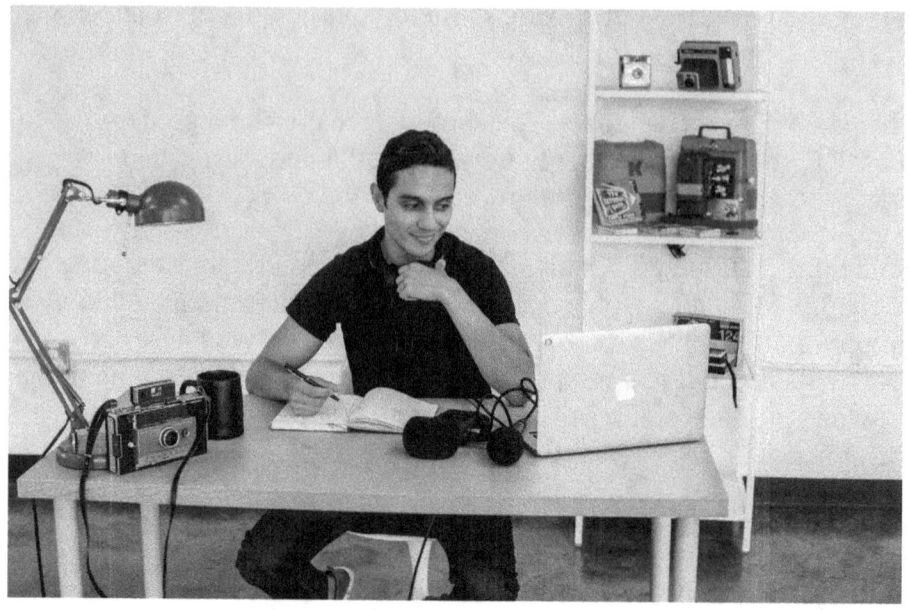

Have you heard the quote by Benjamin Franklin: *"by failing to prepare, you are preparing to fail"*?

This is so true.

But why is this important?

You need to always know the locations/ business you want new patients from ahead of time. This way you know the exact strategies to use when it comes to Ground Marketing.

For example, in the Ground Marketing Course we have many strategies. It wouldn't make sense for you to use the Restaurant Strategy on Apartments. These are two different kinds of businesses! No one strategy works for every single business.

Also, you don't want to blindly try and get into a business, spend a ton of time and energy getting in, only to figure out that the business you're Ground Marketing too only has employees that want the cheapest and lowest price in town (unless you want to be that dentist)!

You also can't just go out and drop off freebies and hope people will see the freebies and call you to make an appointment.

THIS IS **NOT** GROUND MARKETING!

You need to know why you are wanting to visit these specific locations/ businesses.

Maybe you want to get into these businesses because they have great dental insurance, or maybe they have no dental insurance, or maybe they are high income earners... whatever the case is... you need to know who to talk with, what to present, what to say, and how to attract the right patients from this business to your practice.

So, *preparation is key!*

You need to ALWAYS be strategic with your Ground Marketing. So how can you do that? How can you be specific and strategic with your Ground Marketing?

You need to create something we call a "Starter List" first!

STEP TWO: *Create Your Starter List.*

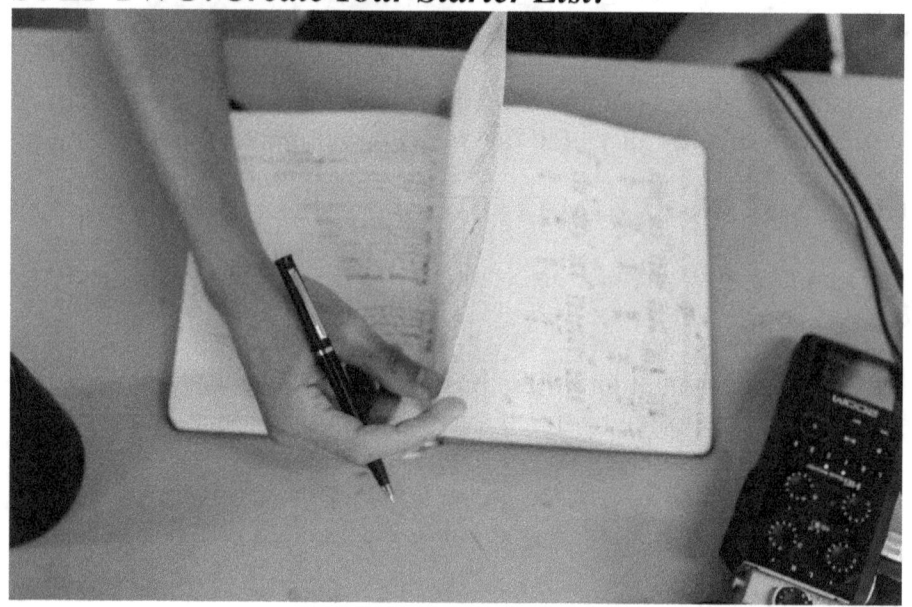

What I want you to do is gather together with your team (or it could just be you too) and start brainstorming.

You need to brainstorm on the type of patients you want in your practice. If you have existing patients, think about your favorite patients...

Where do they work?

Where do they live?

Are they homeowners or apartment/ loft people?

Do they have kids?

Where do their kids go to school?

Where do they shop?

Do they like coffee?

What coffee shops do they go to?

Think of as many of these questions as you possibly can, brainstorm, and answer them as specific as possible.

If you don't have an existing patient base, still ask yourselves these questions. Ask yourself *"what type of patient do I want in my practice? Where do I want them to be shopping? Where do I want them to live? Where do I want them to work? etc."*

All of the answers to these questions must be accurate and specific locations in your community.

So, don't just say "I want them to live in luxury apartments". I want you to name the luxury apartment complex you are thinking of in your community. That's how specific you need to be.

Once you have the answers to this… now you have a "STARTER LIST".

This list is your guide/ starting point for knowing what businesses/ locations you need to START targeting with your Ground Marketing.

So, for example let's say you said: "my existing patient works at a WELLS FARGO BANK".

Write "WELLS FARGO" down. This is one business you will be Ground Marketing too! Wells Fargo is now on your "Starter List".

Then you move on to the next question.

"Does my existing patient love coffee?… Yes! They do!...What coffee shop does he/she go too?... Hmmm I remember seeing a Starbucks cup in their hand so… Starbucks!"

Write down Starbucks on your "Starter List".

Now you are creating a list of the locations you will be Ground Marketing too.

You are starting to have a much better idea of who you are targeting, the types of businesses you are going into, and now you know you will be attracting more of your ideal patients!

Next is our last step…

You need to not only locate the businesses on your Starter List, but you also need to find more similar businesses in a matter of seconds and check to see if they are too far and possibly not worth your efforts and time.

STEP THREE: *Community Research & Radius Checks*

Community Research and Radius Checks help you to LOCATE the businesses on your Starter List and find more similar businesses with great potential!

So, for example, let's say on your Starter List you have written down schools, coffee shops, surgeons, banks, etc.

I want you to expand your list and start thinking of other businesses that are similar but probably a different corporation/ company. For example, let's say on your list you have "Chase Bank"… well why not also put "Wells Fargo Bank" if you know there is a Wells Fargo near you. Continue to do this with all the businesses in your Starter List.

Now, let's find these locations/ businesses and see if they qualify for Ground Marketing!

The way you will locate these businesses, find their numbers/ address, and check to see if they are near you or around your community is by doing what we call Community Research & a Radius Check.

There are basically 3 ways to do this:

1. Community Research on a desktop. Use Google and MapQuest.

2.   Community Research on your smartphone. Use Apple Maps or a smart GPS app.

3.   Drive around your community for about 30 minutes to an hour once or twice a week.

That's it!

This is how you get started with Ground Marketing. You have a full plan now! You have specific businesses you MUST go see and ground market too!

Now, I know you're probably getting pretty excited now and thinking: "Awesome! Now, how do I get into these locations and get these employees/ customers/ residents/ members to become our new patients"!?

No worries… we will get there! Each location has its specific strategies, specific scripts, specific people we must talk to first and so on…

However, if you want to know NOW, if you want to start bringing in new patients immediately, and get all this information along with training videos, templates, scripts, on-going support from me and my team, and more then feel free to check out The Ground Marketing Course found in our website. In the Ground Marketing Course, we cover everything, from learning how to get new patients from schools and gyms, to getting new patients from senior homes and small business.

Now let's jump into strategy and get into Apartment Complexes.

GROUND MARKETING TO APARTMENTS

A question I get asked often is "Michael, how do we find new families who just moved into the community"?

There are multiple ways… but today I want to teach you one way that will produce MAJOR results and LASTING results…

Think about it…

Where is a location where you can find hundreds of people, where you can find families, where you can find NEW families who just moved into the community, and where you are able to talk and show your practice to all of these people at once?

Apartment Complexes!

Attracting new patients consistently from your local apartments can be simple and highly effective!

BUT…

There is a strategy to it.

I don't want you to go into these Apartment Complexes like everyone else and drop off freebies and try and promote your practice… this is NOT what I want you to do.

I want you to do the strategy in this section, that way I know you will get results FOR SURE!

FIRST... DO THIS!

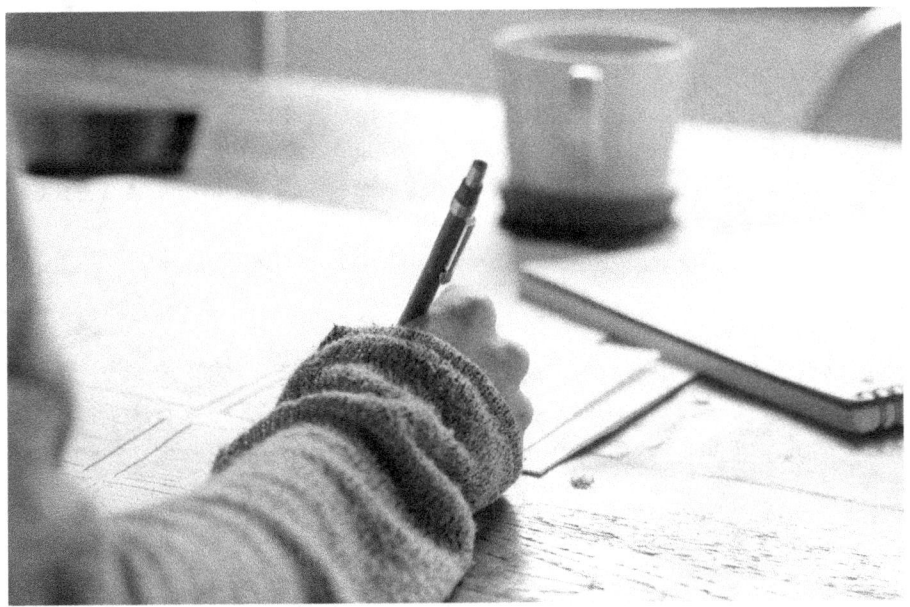

Apartments are FILLED with tons of people who are looking for a great dentist!

Don't believe me?

Just wait and see...

By the end of this you will be doing events, picking up sign-up sheets, and bringing in new patients who want to see you from your local Apartments!

Now, I personally feel everyone should be targeting apartments in your community.

And no, not the way most people do it, which is by leaving door hangers or flyers at the door.

You are actually going to be able to speak to the residents.

Let me give you a run-down of what you will actually be learning in this section:

1. How To Participate in New Patient Packets.
2. How To Walk Into An Apartment Complex and Participate in Their Events.
3. How To Get The Employees from Apartment Complexes To Come In.
4. How To Create a Pipeline with Apartment Complexes so They Continue to FeedYou New Patients!

Now... what I want you to do is...

Take a look around your community.

Start keeping an eye out for apartment complexes that you would like to target.

Write down *5 Apartment Complexes* you would like to Ground Market to.

If you decide to make a bigger list (more than 5) then that's awesome!

Make the list as big as you'd like but it has to have a minimum of 5 Apartment Complexes.

Then... get ready... because we are going to be Ground Marketing to these locations on your list!

OPERATION: LET'S GET INTO THESE APARTMENTS!

Now that you have your list of Apartment Complexes you will be visiting... it's time to get into them!

This strategy will NOT be done over the phone. This strategy involves you WALKING INTO the Apartment Complex.

This also means you need to do research and see what days and times they are open. You do not want to go to an Apartment Complex... pull up... and then realize it's closed.

I don't want you to waste time.

So just Google Search the apartment complex. Then either click on maps and find the apartments you want to get into and see the times they close and open.

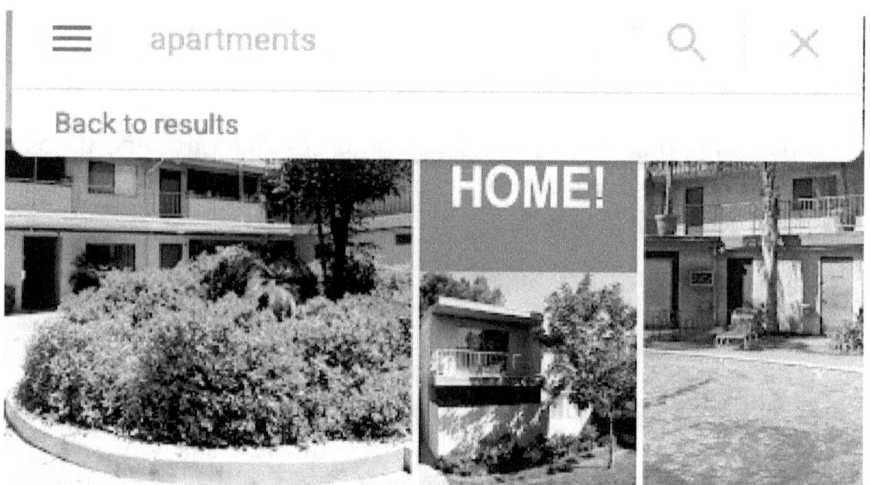

Mission Village

3.0 ★ ★ ★ ★ ★ (15)

Apartment building

 Directions   Save   Nearby   Send to your phone   Share

📍   154 N Palmetto Ave, Ontario, CA 91762

⋮⋮   387J+XQ Ontario, California

🌐   missionvillageontario.com

📞   (909) 986-4417

🕐   Closed. Opens at 10:00 AM ∨

🏷   Add a label

Once you have done that... now it's time to start heading out to these apartments!

Here is the strategy and script you will say once you walk into the apartment complex:

When you go visit the Apartment Complex, you want to walk-in with NOTHING in hand. Just walk in and use the script:

You: Hello!

Them: Hello!

You: I was wondering if you guys distribute NEW MOVE-IN PACK-ETS?

THEM: yes/ no/ we should.

You: (if they say YES) oh awesome! I'm actually with the dental of-fice right here (point in that location) and wanted to see if we could have our information in your NEW MOVE-IN PACKETS?

Them: YES!

You: Ok awesome! I actually have some gift certificates/ flyers in the car, if that's ok? I can just go get them really quick.

Them: YEAH!

You: (go to the car.. get the flyers)

You: (give them flyers) and then say: I also wanted to give you and the employees here (an incentive that is one the sign-up sheet) if that's ok with you?

THEM: of course it is!!

You: Wonderful! When should I come back to pick up the sign-up sheet?

THEM: (tells you date and time)

You: Wonderful! I'll also come back with new move-in flyers. I also wanted to know... by any chance do you guys do any events for the residents?

THEM: (if they say YES)

You: Oh cool! Do you think we could ever participate and like set-up a small booth and give ALL the residents here free hygiene kits? Like toothbrushes, paste, mouthwash, floss and more?

THEM: Yes of course!

You: (Schedule a date and time you can participate at their event AND don't forget to come back and pick up the sign-up sheet as well)

That's it!

A couple pointers I want you to keep in mind is:

1. Be Casual. Don't walk in there with clipboards, a gift basket, pamphlets, and you in a suit. You need to be as casual as possible. A good example is just pretending like you were walking by after lunch and said to yourself *"hey since I'm here, might as well check this place out"*. Have a coffee in hand if possible! That's how casual I need you to be.

2. Don't give them 100s of flyers. Just give them around 10 for their new move in packets. If they tell you "this is to little" then that's fine... when you come back to pick up the sign-up sheet you can always bring more. This goes along with our next point.

3. Remember, you are building a pipeline, a relationship with this

Apartment Complex. You want consistent new patients coming from here. Consistent referrals. So treat them well and they will do the same in return.

Some start-ups I have worked with have built a huge part of their patients base off of Ground Marketing to Apartments alone!

Just imagine... if you did this strategy with every... single... apartment complex in your community!

You and I both know the results will be tremendous!

Now that you know an amazing strategy that WILL get you new patients, I want you to execute and do it.

I don't just want you bookmarking this section or saving it for later. I want you to see the results!

Go out and execute!

Let me know the results!

Finally, I want to discuss a topic I have been seeing on many forums.

Right now, we are experiencing a world wide pandemic and there is an uprising in the case numbers.

Social distancing has caused us to pivot a bit, to change things up with how you interact with people, and it has caused us to limit ourselves.

Many of the people in your community are still skeptical to go out to events, parties, gatherings (but somehow everyone is ok to gather at Target and Costco -_-).

I want you to remember that this does not damper your Grand Opening Party, or your Open House, or even any event that you had plan to throw in your practice.

Instead this has caused you to save a bit more money, to think outside the box, and to stay safe!

You can still, definitely, do a Grand Opening Party/ Open House!

Let me show you what I am talking about!

How To Do a Grand Opening/ Open House During COVID-19

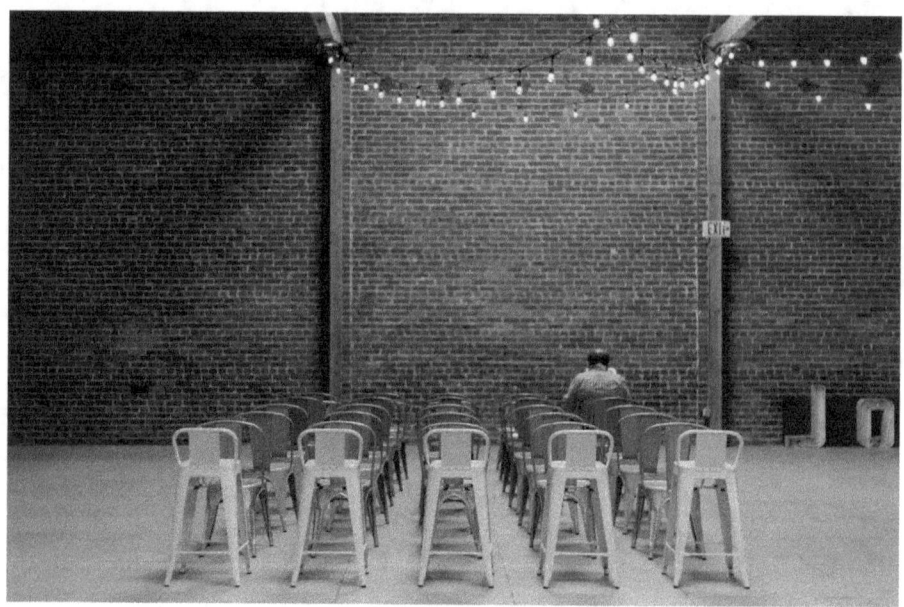

What Are You Going To Do?

First things first, we need to decide if this is going to be an "IN-PERSON" Event OR a Virtual Event.

In this section I will talk about the pros and cons of both during the pandemic.

IN-PERSON EVENT

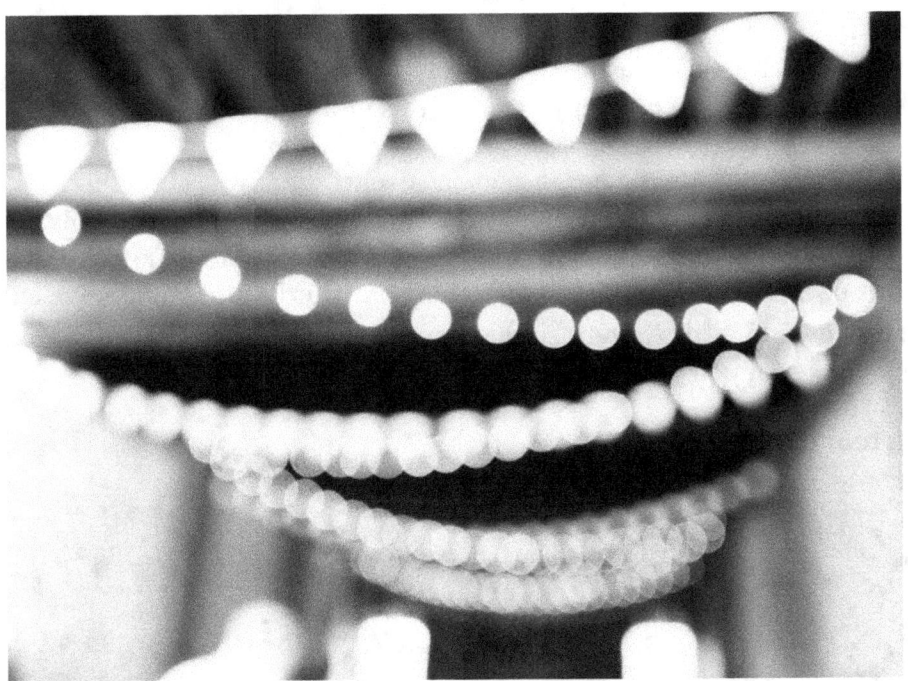

This is obviously the best move, if there was no virus going around.

However, since there is a pandemic currently happening (November 2020), an "in-person" event would have to be much more controlled and much more private. If you do plan to throw a "in-person" event, then I recommend a couple things:

- Make it exclusive.

- Make it fancy.

- Broadcast it virtually.

I recommend only doing an "in-person" grand opening/ event for family and friends OR for the community influencers only.

Keep it small and reasonable according to your community/ state's guidelines.

The CONS for throwing this type of event is that you are running a risk, you can get backlash from people (depending on how many people you invite at once), and you can spend more time and money.

The PROS for throwing an "in-person" event is you will get influencers and friends in your actual space. Create stronger connections. You can get content of people being in your practice and enjoying the atmosphere. You can get others opinions on your location, and you can easily invite 5 "VIPs" every single hour and broadcast the office tour or their journey in your practice as a new patient.

Virtual Events

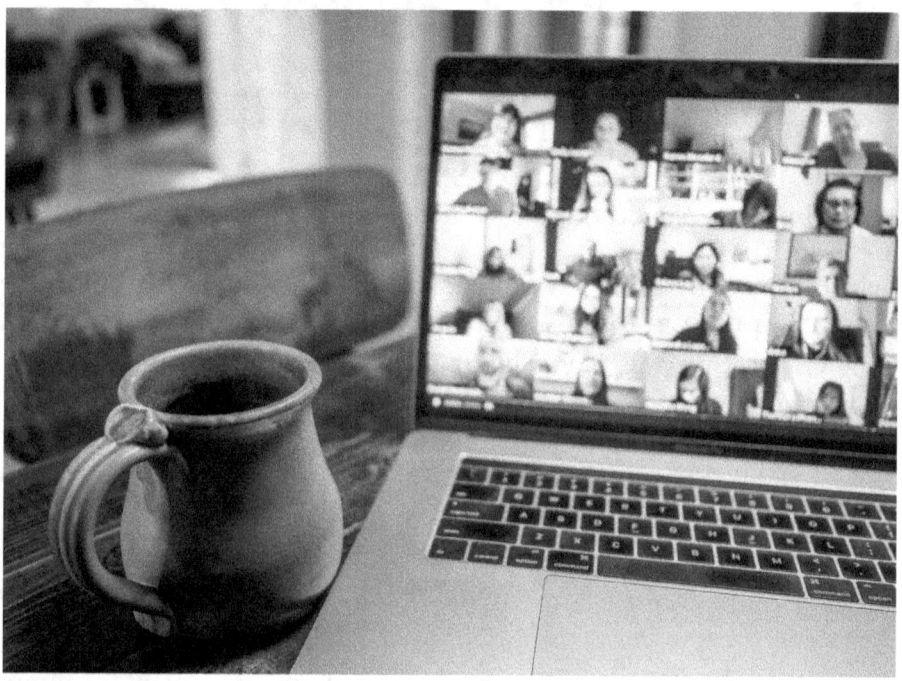

Virtual Events are exciting and can have many possibilities!

You can invite as many people as you desire or continue to keep it exclusive. This is less personable, obviously, but you are still showing your community how your practice looks and functions... and you are still doing a "Grand Opening" / "Open House" event.

The PROs of doing a Virtual Event is the risk level of attending comes down to zero!

You are hosting it in your practice and you don't have to worry about it getting out of hand. You are also saving tons of money by doing this. You are able to invite more people. Much more opportunities for people to share it all over social media/ online. You can still do giveaways, prizes, office tours, and introductions of your team.

The CONs are minimal but very important. Your internet connection can be unstable or go down. If you are using ZOOM, everyone can be talking over everyone and they won't be able to hear you (this is why you will need someone doing the operations and muting everyone and then allowing people to speak/ participate when it is time for them to do so). You need to be 100x more organized with your itinerary and how you will run the Virtual Event.

The Virtual Event needs to feel like a party.

Don't plan it to be hours and hours long. It's ok if your Virtual Event looks like this:

Grand Opening Party

Starts at 7pm. Say "HI" introduce your practice and why you started in THIS community. Also mention how there will be prizes for them at the end of the party (so stick around)!

7:05pm Introduce Team Members

7:10pm Office Tour

Ask everyone to virtually raise their hand if they have any questions about the team or the office tour (plan out 5 minutes just in case, if no one raises their hand, continue).

7:15pm Introduce a "FREEBIE" like "Free Exams" for everyone attending this event. Show them where they can sign-up (LocalMed, on your website, or let them know to enter their email in the chat section). Make sure you pin in the chat section ways to contact you (phone, email, website, social media, etc.).

7:20pm Thank all the businesses who participated in contributing to the giveaway and mention all the prizes! Hype it up!

7:25pm Let people know one last time that they can enter in the raffle to win prizes by simply going to your Social Media, make sure they follow you and liking the post, if they share the post/ party then they will get 5 more tickets for their raffle. While you wait for people to do this you can play a quick Virtual Game or say hi to absolutely everyone by name and thank them for joining/ attending.

7:26pm Start the raffle and name the winners! If they won ask them to virtually raise their hand. Make it a big deal with each prize winner, ask for their email/ contact info so they can pick up the prizes.

7:40pm Thank everyone, remind them about how everyone who attended will be able to redeem their free exam within the month (30 day period). All they have to do is put their email address in the chat and one of your team members will reach out.

7:42pm Unmute everyone and play music and say goodbye! Have your whole team sit there and wave. Literally you and your team can wave for a whole 2 minutes until you start seeing a majority of people leaving. Once a majority of people leave you can choose to end the event or stay on and talk more, it's up to you.

What you can also do is let them know (before you unmute everyone and say goodbye), if they want to see behind the scene stuff and more of what is happening in the virtual event (maybe you invited the media, influencers, or other partners) then go over to your Instagram or Facebook and see what's happening! Let them know how the party is still going on there!

That's all you have to do in a Virtual Event! You don't have to make it an hour long even! Keep it simple, impactful, make sure there is no "dead-air" or long silences, and keep it going!

You can always do a HYBRID version as well.

Invite some local influencers and do the major Virtual Event as well. You can still keep it controlled and exciting this way.

Now that you have decided what type of event you want to do, let's talk about how we can market it.

FOUR WAYS TO MARKET YOUR GRAND OPENING DURING COVID-19

1. Start Ground Marketing (safely).

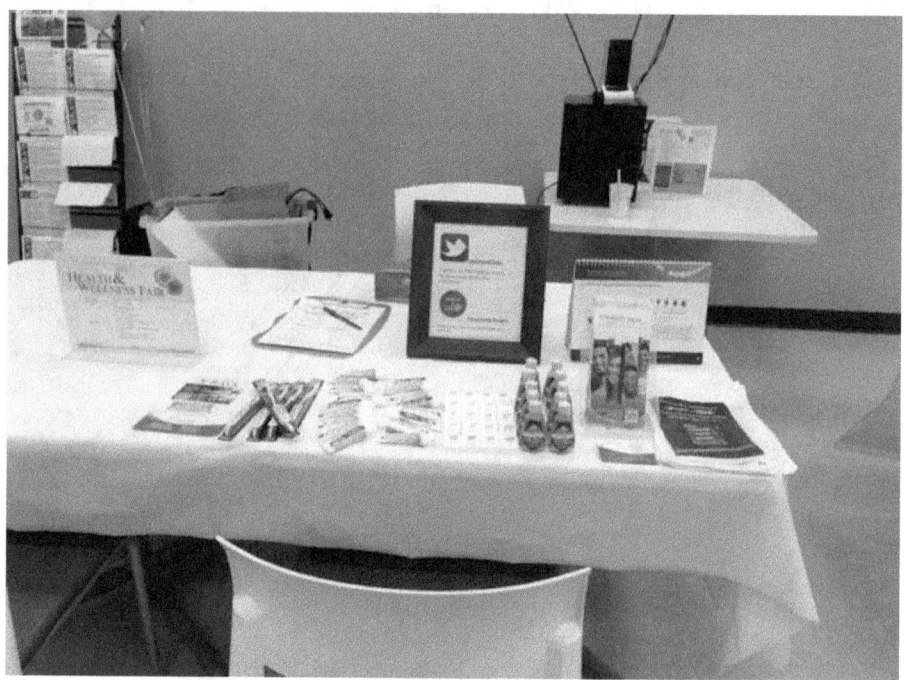

You're not alone in this COVID-19 struggle. All businesses are learning how to adapt, pivot, and stay above water. Be the helping hand here.

Even if you and other businesses are only operating at a limited capacity, it doesn't mean you can't come together with others in your local neighborhood to create some positive support for the community.

You need to start letting other businesses in your shopping strip or community know that you are going to be opening up soon!

How should you let them know?

You can drop by and do the age old thing where you say:

"Hey! Just wanted to give you cookies and let you know we are opening soon and accepting new patients! Here is our info."

You walk away.

This may FEEL like you are doing *good* ground marketing but it's really not doing as much as you feel or think it is.

Instead do this:

Walk in with nothing in hand and say-

"Hey! I was wondering if I could have some of your information?"

They will ask *"why"*?

You will say *"I am from the brand new dental office down the street and we are doing a Grand Opening and I wanted to have some of your info on hand to display to our visitors AND if you have any amazing deals or giveaways for prizes we can definitely have that too"*!

They will be ecstatic! They will want to participate!

Once they tell you *"great let me go get some info etc."*, then you want to invite them to your grand opening!

If it's a Virtual Event then extend the invite to them and also let them know that they can invite their family, friends, and customers. If they gave you a prize/ deal to giveaway as a prize, let them know that you will be announcing the prize during the Virtual Event. Encourage them to share this on their social media for more exposure.

Once you have collected their information, thank them and invite them to come to your office so they can check it out. Call it a "private tour". During the "private tour" you can schedule them for an appointment/ exam. Let them know how you can take a picture of them at your practice and tag them on your social media so your followers can see it.

This means more exposure for your practice and their company as well!

Do this with every single business possible.

2. Contact Your Local Chamber of Commerce/ Rotary Club

Reach out to the Chamber of Commerce and ask them if you could participate or host an event.

Believe it or not, this is still happening! Your local chamber of commerce and rotary clubs are still hosting tons of events and ribbon cuttings! Some may be "in-person" events but the majority are Virtual Events.

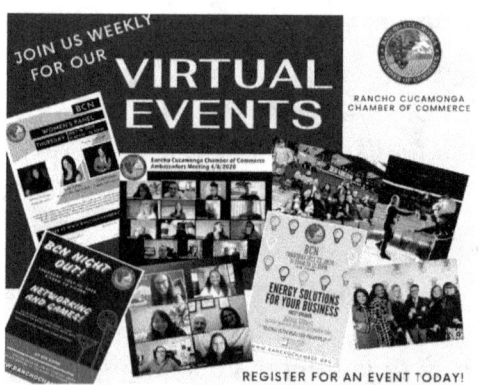

Just take a look:

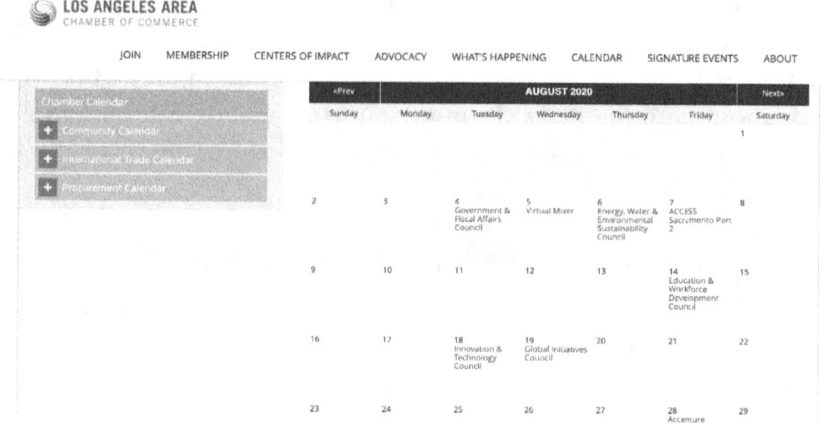

3. Invite the Local News

We are ALL starving for some amazing, good news. Local newspapers and television stations are looking for a positive story, which includes your grand opening.

Don't be shy about inviting the press because it's a free opportunity to market your practice! Make sure you leave no attempts/ opportunities on the table!

This means I want you to reach out to and invite print media, radio media, television, and even any local podcasters.

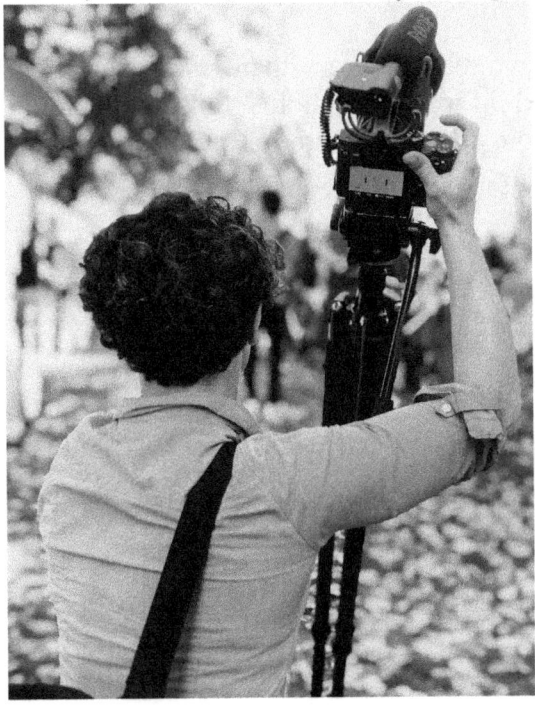

Here are a few tips when attracting news coverage for your grand opening:

" **Make your grand opening news-friendly:** Will there be something interesting to video? Do you have a special occurrence planned, such as an appearance by a local celebrity/ influencer or a live demonstration? If so, be sure to provide a schedule of events.

Invite and remind: As soon as you know your grand opening date, send a short message to get on news professionals' radar. For newspapers, forward a full press release about a week before the event. For radio and TV, send the press release 24 to 48 hours before the event. The day before the event, call and email reporters to ask if they are attending.

Create a Grand Opening Press Release: Include the 5 Ws — who, what, where, when, and why — and a quote from you about the event. Write the press release as if it would appear directly in the newspaper. Reporters will often your exact words from the press release you provided.

After the event, be sure to reach out to reporters, thank them for attending, and send any promised information (photos, links, etc.) and even invite them for a free tour/ exam/ procedure for them and their family (remember, you are trying to get new patients)".

4. Document Your Grand Opening Preparation

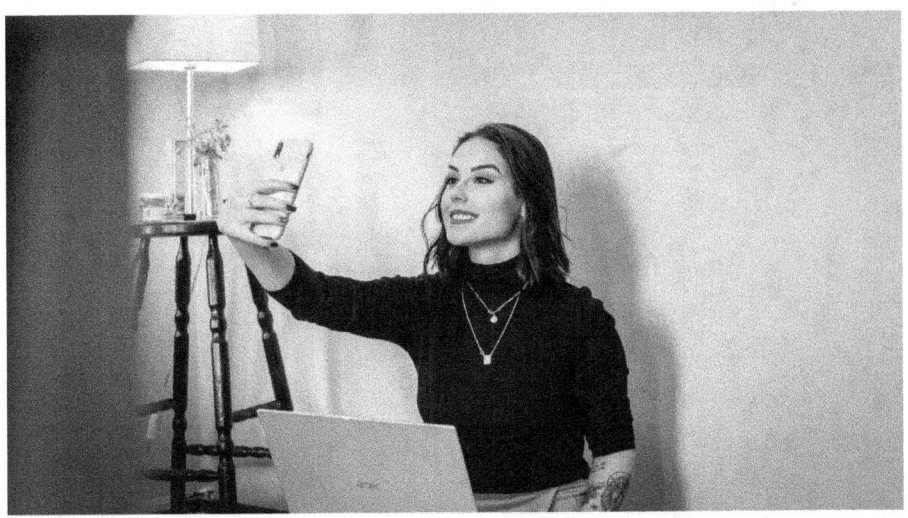

You can document and share your journey to doing a Grand Opening!

This can mean everything from taking photos, talking about your vision of the Grand Opening/ Open House, sharing videos of your staff preparing, etc.

This kind of content not only lets your community know that you'll be opening soon, but it can also help to soothe some of their anxieties about visiting the dentist or your practice during COVID-19.

A recent Nielsen study shows that 50% of consumers want to see social distancing accommodations and 49% are looking for additional hygiene programs/ protocols. If you can show consumers that you're taking extra steps to keep them safe, it can help to make them feel more comfortable.

5. Announce on Facebook & Instagram (there's actually a section for this on Facebook).

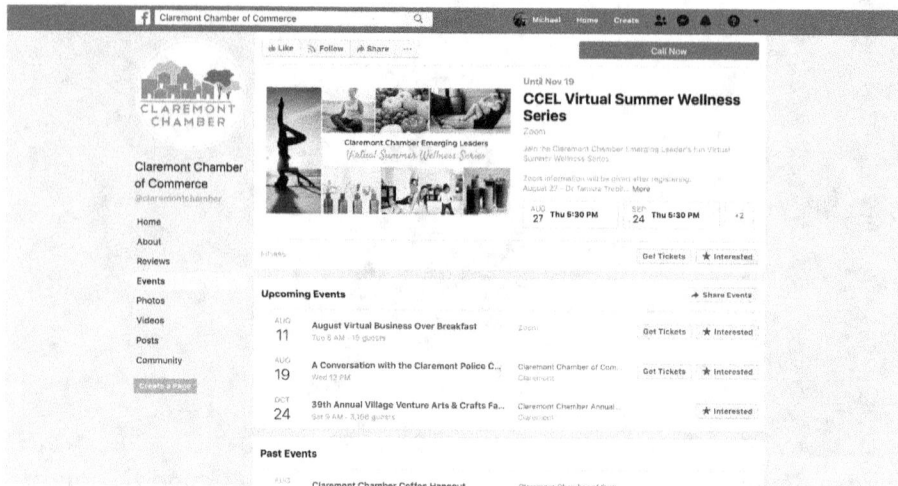

There are thousands of other businesses doing events virtually and they are announcing it on their Social Media!

A Facebook event page is a free and easy-to-setup way to advertise your Grand Opening. Honestly, even if there was no pandemic, this should be part of your marketing. It's especially useful if you already have a following on a Facebook group or fan page.

When creating your event page, be sure to include images and videos that make the event appealing. Also, include anything special like prizes, live music, grand opening specials, or discounts. Once you have the event page link, promote it on social media, through your newsletter, or with Facebook or Instagram.

As you get closer to the event, add posts on the event page with more information about:

- Product and services highlights
- Personal messages about why you and your employees are excited for the grand opening
- Event teasers to build excitement

- A branded hashtag—so it's easier to collect photos from those who attend the event.

So... what are some good giveaways/ party favors/ freebies you can give during your Grand Opening/ Open House?

WHAT TO GIVEAWAY?

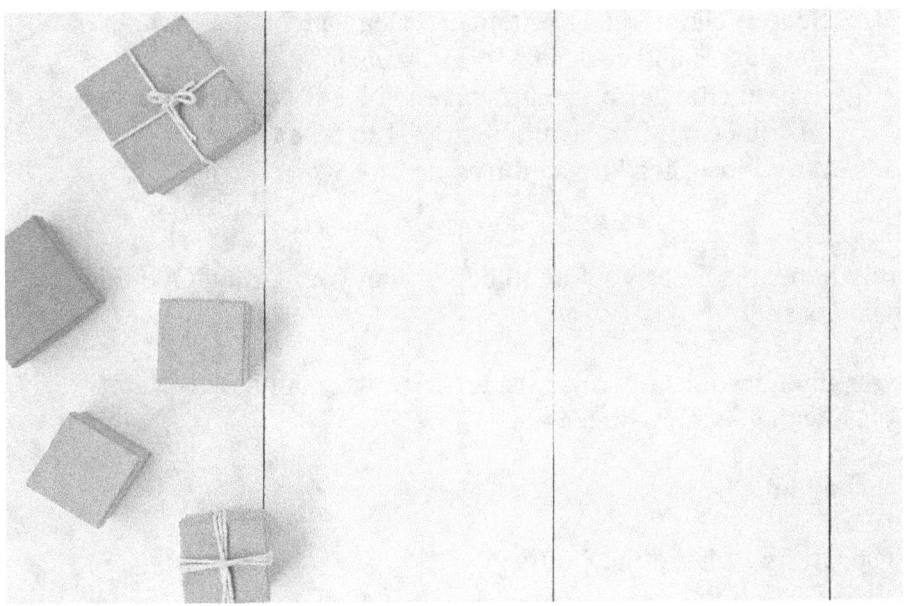

Try something unique, useful during these times, and something that is related to your industry/ brand.

You will NEVER go wrong with giving away "hygiene kits". Especially in times like this where "hygiene" is extremely important.

I do NOT recommend you give the same old boring giveaways like: pens, magnets, cups and stickers. Everyone is doing that, they are barely useful and not unique or memorable.

Try these ideas (if you decide to do more than "hygiene kits") :

- **Branded face masks:** A useful gift that costs around $1 to $2.50 apiece to create
- **Ear savers:** A more affordable alternative to face masks that cost from 50 cents to $1 a piece
- **Travel hand sanitizers:** Customize the bottle with your logo with a cost from $.75 to $2 per bottle
- **Laptop webcam covers:** This item provides reassurance when people are using their laptops and cost anywhere from $.10 to $.75 a piece
- **Screen cleaners:** This item can clean a tech item screen or sunglasses and cost $.15 to $1.50 each
- **Travel chargers:** An attractive choice if you have high-tech customers and are available for $1 to $5 each
- **Any "in-office" procedures.**

I truly hope this helps you out to better plan your Grand Opening/ Open House!

If you any questions or concerns, feel free to email me at michael@thedentalmarketer.site

You can find:

- The Ground Marketing Course

- The Pediatric Dental Marketing Course

- Listen to The Dental Marketer Podcast

- Read extremely helpful dental marketing strategies and articles

- See videos of me actually executing the apartment strategy and more here:

www.thedentalmarketer.org

References:

My Own Experience

https://fitsmallbusiness.com/grand-opening-marketing/

https://fitsmallbusiness.com/

https://www.touchbistro.com/

You can download the Starter List, **Content**

Chapter 8
Human Resources 101
The Class that was missing in your dental education

By: Samantha Leonard, CEO and Co-Founder Stream Dental HR
&
Olivia Robertson, GPHR, CPHR, SHRM-SCP HR Strategist with Stream Dental HR

You are reading this book because you want to do 'starting a dental practice' right!

You have done all the arduous work; you have secured your funding, you found the perfect location, you have been approved for your insurance, you have built your brand and have your marketing and advertising materials ready to go!

Word then spreads around the neighborhood and your patient base starts to grow to the point where you don't have enough hours in the day to meet the demand! WOOHOO!

But can you continue to run this practice (the practice of your dreams!) as a one person show?!

Probably not.

It's expansion time! Time to bring on more team members and build your tribe as you form a team that supports your business vision while keeping the integrity of your services.

Suddenly you are not just managing physical resources, you are managing _human_ resources.

But now the systems, processes, and "ways of doing things" no longer work. The bottlenecks and drama within your office is increasing and suddenly so are your headaches as well.

You spend your life convincing people that the Dentist is not scary and meanwhile you are starting to feel a little scared of going to work every day. That's not right and that's not how it should be.

Suddenly, you are more than just a Dentist.

You are now a business owner, CEO, and an HR manager.

In between seeing patients, you were learning how to manage and run a business because that was not part of your education in dental school.

You find yourself jumping in between roles and tasks that you end up operating your practice from a state of reactivity, instead of being proactive. Without your HR standards, policies, and procedures in place, you are now spending at least one third of a new hire's annual salary on every employee replacement you make due to having high turnover rates.

Instead of working on your business vision to scale into adding new services, bring on an associate, or expand to new locations, you were spending time trying to manage bad employees while living through the repetitious pattern of what feels like Groundhog Day. Nothing kills your passion for being a dentist quicker than working with the wrong people. And the biggest tragedy is your patients start to feel your practice slip, they start to cancel, no-show, or worse...take their business to your competitor for treatment instead! You should look forward to coming to your office – not dread it!

So how do you prevent this from happening? How do you keep your vision alive and fight off the HR nightmares that are haunting the dreams so many dental practice owners around the world?

A common theme that you will continue to see over the entirety of this chapter (and the entire book!) is the importance of setting yourself up correctly from the very moment you start your business as this will make your life exponentially easier as you grow and hire more employees in the future. While it is time consuming and requires some investment to set the stage correctly from the inception of your practice, the savings you will continue to have over time will save you not only financially, but also emotionally and physically.

There are few things more stressful to an employer than the threat of an impending lawsuit – especially when you honestly did not know you were doing anything wrong. This will eat at your finances, your emotional health, and will likely cause you to develop physical stress responses as well. *(Trust us - been there, done that!)*

Why is it important to lay out the worst-case-scenarios when it comes to HR?

Because we are all about risk mitigation.

HR is a direct business function that protects both the employees of an organization, and their employer, from having to go through the unnecessary stress, and financial toll that develops as an outcome from issues stemming from a lack of compliance. We do not write this to scare you – but instead, we write this to **inform you**, because we believe that knowledge is power and that you deserve to know what *could* happen if you do not focus on setting up your HR correctly from the start.

Think of HR as if you are buying a house – specifically a fixer-upper. Is it easier to renovate and remodel the house before you move all your furniture and personal belongings in, or later? Obviously, the answer is before – but with the caveat that cost must be considered. Did you consider the cost of moving yourself and your family into a hotel and putting your belongings in storage while you renovate later once you have more cash flow?

You want to build the practice of your dreams – would you leave the drywall unpainted before opening and seeing patients? Of course not. So why are you stopping yourself from providing your future team and co-workers with the best foundation for long term growth and professional development within your office?

Furthermore, how do you plan to keep up with your practice as time goes on? If a computer dies, you replace it. If the hydraulics in your chair are on the fritz, you call your technician. If your plumbing is not working correctly, you call your plumber. But what do you do if your team breaks down? You call your HR Professional!

People management is not everyone's favorite topic. It is likely that you went into dentistry for other reasons than to talk to people all day long. However, just because you did not go to school to manage people, does not mean that you are incapable of effectively managing your team! Let us focus on the importance of clear communication and the idea of mutual expectations.

Clear Communication – the Vitality of any Successful Dental Practice

Dr. Tooth opened her practice three months ago and is still in the process of getting to know her team. Dr. Tooth has hired three employees initially (an administrator, assistant and hygienist) to help grow her new practice. During this time, she has noticed that there are discrepancies in how patient charts are kept, how patient files are updated, where certain items are kept within the practice, and that some tasks are completed inconsistently. She has had a team meeting to discuss these issues but has not noticed any improvements yet. What should Dr. Tooth do now?

Clear communication is a concept that is required within every successful interaction within your dental practice. However, it is important to remember that developing clear communication abilities is a skill that takes time to develop. To begin to understand how you can communicate better with your new team, you must ask yourself the following questions:

What does clear communication look like to ME? What am I saying to my team? Is this what I mean?

What does clear communication look like to MY TEAM? Do they understand what I am saying? Do they understand my intentions?

What does clear communication sound like? Can my team relay the information I give to them back to me, and does it align with my intended meaning?

Let us talk about Dr. Tooth's situation here:

In her last staff meeting, Dr. Tooth said, *"I'm noticing that patient charts aren't filled out how I like them to be, the notes are a mess, I can't find the portable eyewash kit, and when was the last time someone took out the garbage?"*

What Dr. Tooth really meant was, *"I notate items differently in the patient charts than my assistant does. We need to create a better charting system and notes that work and will continue to work over the long term as the practice grows. We need to clearly define where items and equipment are meant to be kept and stored so that we all know where to access them when we need them. And we need to review who is responsible for what daily, weekly, and monthly tasks around here so that we can keep up with the required housekeeping and hygiene regulations that are outlined in our OSHA documentation and Infection Prevention Program."*

What Dr. Tooth should say is, *"Let's schedule some one-on-one times where we can review your Key Performing Indicators (KPIs) and really get these systems and processes standardized so that we can support a growing practice as more patients come to us. We need to have these growing pains worked out before we hire more staff members so that you feel confident in training and onboarding new team members as our department leaders. While we are all meeting today, let us review where our moveable items, tools and equipment are stored so that we can determine where the best long-term placement for these items are. And let's go through our house keeping schedule so that we can figure out who is going to be responsible for which tasks on a daily, weekly, and monthly basis. Do you have any questions or feedback for me on how I can make this process smother and more efficient for you?"*

As you can see, the difference between what Dr. Tooth said initially, and what she should have said is the difference that is required to uphold prominent levels of clear communication for your entire team.

Your team will observe how you communicate with them and begin to mirror the behavior back to you and to the rest of your team. This is the purest example of behavior mirroring that is commonly seen within the workplace.

Your team will also learn to communicate better with one another over time as they have more lived experiences with one another. When everything is new, it is difficult (but not impossible) to find shared patterns of communication. You cannot refer to a specific situation, inside joke, or code for something until you have built those communication pathways within the entire team. There are no short-cuts to getting to this point, it just takes time and continued elevated level practice to ensure that you are setting up communication foundations that can be continually supported throughout the growth of your practice.

Moreover, how do you course correct when you see communication is dwindling within your practice? You see employees that are being short with one another based on a miscommunication the previous day, yet you don't know how to fix it. Should you ignore it and let the employees sort it out themselves? Or should you intervene?

As much as it is a nuisance to help to solve the interpersonal issues between two employees, as an employer this is a part of your role until you have a dedicated office manager to take over the 'management' aspects of your role as owner and employer. In these instances, we recommend utilizing conflict de-escalation strategies (such as using "I" statements) to clear the air between these employees. At the end of the day, the sooner you can facilitate a peace treaty between these team members, the sooner you can get back to focusing on your upwards trajectory towards success with a highly functioning team of employees.

Increased effective patient communication is a side benefit of focusing on clear communication strategies (and practicing them – because the ability to communicate clearly is like a muscle that needs a good workout daily!). Not only will focusing on clear communication within the team help to strengthen your employee's morale and rapport with one another and you, but then they will also learn to communicate more effectively with patients which is a win for everybody involved!

Happy patients = Successful team of employees = Thrilled & effacious employer!

Mutual Expectations – People Management's Best Friend

Now Dr. Tooth didn't take our advice and didn't schedule those one-on-one meetings with her team and has continued to see no improvement from her staff. She is frustrated that no matter how many times she tells her staff to fill out the patient charts like she would, there still hasn't been an improvement. The notes are missing key details, information about prescribed treatment, and there is no medical history being updated in their chart (how Dr. Tooth likes it), and there are too many "personal" notes about the patients in the files. How could her assistant be so blind when Dr. Tooth keeps the patient's personal information on a separate area in the patient chart.

Dr. Tooth's assistant, Suzie, on the other hand, has started to write and organize the notes in the charts like Dr. Tooth does and is quite proud of how quickly she caught on to Dr. Tooth's system! Suzie feels that she is improving but is still struggling on getting through the charts as quickly as possible, which is making her late for her next patient. Dr. Tooth is now interviewing for a new assistant (who she thinks requires more attention to detail) and is planning on letting Suzie go. What are the identifiable problems here?

What exactly is a mutual expectation? A mutual expectation is a by-product of clear communication as it clearly describes the expectations of both an employee and an employer in each situation, or how a certain project should be completed with a particular objective or intention in mind.

Let's say it's Monday, and you have asked your administrator to follow up on insurance billings. Stated as such, you are leaving this open ended and up for further interpretation. You might expect this should be completed by the end of the day based on the knowledge that you have of a hard bookkeeping deadline coming up on Wednesday, while your administrator thinks that the end of the week is an appropriate timeline for that project. Then Thursday rolls around and you've asked your administrator why this isn't complete after you got a call from your bookkeeper last night, and the administrator says they had planned on doing it tomorrow. You're now annoyed because you thought it would be done 3 days ago and you have missed your deadline!

What you said, "Can you follow up on the insurance billings ASAP?"

What you meant, "I want you to prioritize these and have them done by the end of today because we have a hard deadline of Wednesday for our bookkeeping purposes"

What you should have said, "I know things have been busy, but I need you to put everything aside at this point and just focus on the insurance billings. They need to be completed today, so that our bookkeeper has time to review them tomorrow to not impact our hard deadline of Wednesday. Does that make sense? Is that possible? What can the team do to support you so that we can ensure this is done by our deadlines?"

As much as an employer is technically a "boss," the employment relationship is still not entirely unilateral. There needs to be some give and take, and this is where mutual expectations really come into play. To create a dedicated team that genuinely loves their work and who they work with (including you, their employer!), they need to know what to expect from the people around them, and what the people around them expect from them! It all works full circle here to support a workplace that is full of expert communicators.

Moreover, people want to be good at their jobs and want to be effective team players within their workplace. Most people don't show up to work with the intention of doing a poor job and are usually quite disappointed when they find out their employers don't think that they are doing a wonderful job either. To ensure that your team is full of awesome employees, you need to help them to be the best forms of themselves by providing them with clear expectations that are appropriate and manageable for all parties involved.

Your employees won't come to work with the sole intention of making you miserable (unless they're reciprocating what you are doing to them), therefore we want to respect the golden rule! We are going to treat our team with fair expectations and give them an opportunity to provide us feedback when they feel that they are overwhelmed, and in turn we are going to maintain whatever standards we set that our employees can depend on us for.

Performance management is also guided by proper usage of mutual expectations. If there is a gap in the knowledge, skills or abilities (KSAs) of your team members, this is likely due to a lack of communication or mutual expectation in what was presented in the employee's job description initially, and then what your team members were trained to do during the orientation, getting acquainted or probationary period. If you feel like your team is letting you down, take a step back and see where the miscommunication has developed from.

Sometimes employees are not always a good fit for a specific job or the culture of a workplace. However, most times you will be able to find a crack in your system that the employee slipped through and be able to provide them with some informal coaching to get them up to the standards that you expect from your team in the practice of your dreams. Keep working on clearly communicating these expectations and creating mutual expectations between yourself and your growing team!

Now that you understand the concepts of clear communication and mutual expectations, what should Dr. Tooth do in her situation?

A) Terminate Suzie once a new assistant has been hired. She is an at-will employee and has only been with her for 4 months. Not much damage has been done in Dr. Tooth's mind.

B) Initiate a one-on-one meeting with Suzie. Pull out the assistant's job description and review the knowledge, skills and abilities required to successfully be employed in this position. Ask Suzie why she has not made any improvements after Dr. Tooth has asked her to improve many times. Find out where the lack of mutual expectations is and unpack those issues until a mutual agreement can be made.

C) Don't do anything. Dr. Tooth is too busy trying to see as many pa-tients as she can, and she is absolutely swamped. Her annoyance with Suzie is growing but perhaps she will figure out what Dr. Tooth wants in another few weeks

Answer:

It seems so plain and simple when the answer is laid out on paper. Obviously in this situation, B is the best answer for the situation as it gives the assistant, Suzie, some time to talk to Dr. Tooth about how excited she is about learning Dr. Tooth's notation system and how ready she is to learn more! Hopefully at this point Dr. Tooth will re-member the importance of clear communication and the creation of well-defined mutual expectations so that this employee can improve at an exponentially faster rate than before!

So now that you understand how to effectively communicate with your team to keep them content, productive and loyal, how do you find the best people for the job?

The Employee Life Cycle – Recruitment, Onboarding, Management, Offboarding

Recruitment 101 – The Right People. In the Right Place. At the Right Time.

Dr. Tooth had a good meeting with Suzie, and they uncovered during this meeting that Suzie's workload is growing exponentially with the influx of new patients they have started to see in the last three months. They are gaining a great reputation, which is fantastic for speedy growth for the practice, but the team is exhausted and barely able to keep up with Dr. Tooth's increasingly high-quality demands. The team has been conferring without Dr. Tooth and they are worried that they are going to start making mistakes and ruin all the positive momentum and growth that they have worked so hard with Dr. Tooth to create since the office opened. The team has decided to bring this issue to Dr. Tooth's attention at their weekly meeting on Friday this week and let her know that their capabilities are completely maxed out.

This situation that Dr. Tooth is in is a fantastic sign of success that is wrapped in the disguise of a problem. In this case, the team is feeling the strain of the immense growth that has happened over a brief period. They are maxed out with their capabilities and responsibilities and have the internal acuity to acknowledge that this inconvenience has the potential to turn into a HUGE problem if not attended to carefully.

When it comes to the start of the employee life cycle, you need to focus on not just getting the right people into the right positions, but also the timing of the placement of these individuals. It is worthless to hire an office manager when you do not have employees that need to be managed yet. While having a specific hygiene coordinator might be beneficial in the future, would you benefit more now from someone who can work as an administrator and then transition into a more specific role in the future as you grow? Do you need a lead dental assistant when you only have two assistants to begin with? Or should you wait until your team is larger and start with a clinical lead supervisor?

These are the questions that you must ask yourself as you determine who needs to be hired first, for what role, and at what threshold or capacity? What new hire is going to take the most work off the rest of your team's plate so that they can still uphold your high-level expectations, while also simultaneously training a new team member?

The recruitment process can be broken into nine phases:

Planning for recruitment – where you determine who should be hired, when they should be hired, and what you can afford/what will bring the biggest ROI to your growing practice.

Creation of documents – create your job descriptions, interview questions (specifically for knowledge, skills, abilities, and culture alignment), reference check authorizations, reference check questions, background check authorizations, skills assessment questions, skill assessment authorizations, offer letter, confidentiality agreement, and employment agreement (if applicable).

Job postings – create your job posting, determine where you will post, your budget for the posting, and how much information you wish to disclose.

Resume screenings – determine what you are specifically looking for within a candidate resume (years of experience, certain level of education, skills or additional training and certificates).

Initial phone screenings – ensure that your questions are both legal and lawful to ask and determine how these questions will determine who is going to be a good fit for the role within your office.

In person interviews – ensure that your questions are both legal and lawful to ask, and have all the required documentation ready to sign for the next phase if you will be conducting a skills assessment

Skills Assessments (if applicable) – understand the difference between a skills assessment and a working interview and the requirements of each. Skills assessments are recommended over working interviews to reduce the amount of employer liability that is taken on during these events.

Reference Checks & Background Screenings – ensure that the candidate has signed the appropriate authorization forms for reference checks and/or background screenings, and make sure that all questions asked during a reference check are both legal and lawful.

Offer of Employment – Once the candidate's reference checks and/or background screenings have come back successful you may offer this candidate a position with your practice! Ensure that you have your documentation ready to go from offer letters to confidentiality agreements to employment agreements (if an agreement is necessary for a specific role).

As you can see, the recruitment process is more than just posting a job advertisement and having an employee in place the next day. It takes time, persistence, and requires the employer to have clear expectations and requirements of the position before a new hire starts their first day at your practice.

Dr. Tooth's team told her on Friday that they are feeling extremely maxed out with their workload and Dr. Tooth agreed that she could see their quality of care and attention to detail slipping. The team worked together to determine where they needed the most help and Dr. Tooth agreed that this is the next position that should be filled. Dr. Tooth, with her administrator's help, began the nine-phase recruitment process and found a candidate that they thought would be a perfect fit for the practice.

But then what happens after the recruitment process is completed? This is where the onboarding process begins and will continue forward throughout the employee's first year of employment.

Onboarding – Getting Acquainted and Staying Acquainted

Contrary to widely held belief, the onboarding process is not complete after the employee's first three months of employment. It continues onwards for months past that point until an employee is completely integrated into the workplace.

As you can see from the information provided within this chapter, documentation is key to compliance. During the onboarding process you will proceed through your new hire's orientation, training, initial performance assessments, all the way to their first anniversary of employment with your practice.

The onboarding process can be broken down into eleven phases:

Preparing for the employees first day – there are many documents that the new hire should be signing on their first day (including wage deduction authorizations, safety policies, new hire personal employee information, tax withholding forms, direct deposit authorization forms) and preparing the employee's equipment and other information (key to the office, access codes, passwords, system access, uniforms, locker, PPE, etc.)

New Employee Day 1 – provide the new hire with a tour of the office, introduce the new hire to the rest of the team, have the new hire sign the appropriate documents and acquire the equipment that they need to do their job, introduce the new hire to their direct report and who they will be shadowing, show the new team member an overview of the training documents and materials they will be going through during their first week, have a team lunch/meeting and conduct some icebreaker games.

New Employee Day 2 – begin to review the employee training files and have the new hire job shadow their supervisor/trainer.

New Employee Day 3 – meet with the new hire to review KSAs again and give them the opportunity to ask questions.

New Employee Day 5 – meet with the new hire to get their feedback on how the onboarding process is going so far, ask what questions they have, and meet with the new hire's supervisor/trainer to get direct feedback on how the new hire is integrating into their role.

New Employee Day 15 – meet with the new hire to discuss their performance thus far, review any questions they have, meet with their supervisor/trainer, and discuss where improvements need to be made.

New Employee Day 30 – conduct the first portion of the probationary period review and have the new hire conduct a self-rating on their required competencies and have the supervisor/trainer provide a rating on all required competencies as well as provide some ideas on how to improve performance moving forward.

New Employee Day 60 – conduct the second portion of the probationary period review and have the new hire conduct a self-rating on all their required competencies and have their supervisor/trainer provide a rating on all required competencies as well as provide some ideas on how to improve performance moving forward. Discuss with the new hire what improvements need to be seen to successfully make it through the probationary period after 90 days/three months of employment. You should also see improvements in both the self-ratings and supervisor/trainer ratings of performance for the new hire between the first and second portions of the probationary period reviews.

New Employee Day 90 – this is the point where you will need to decide if this employee will be terminated, continue an unofficial "extended" probationary period, or if they have successfully made it through the probationary period in full. **If you are wishing to extend the probationary period – please check with your state legislation to determine your ability to do so.**

New Employee 6 Month Anniversary – now it is time for the new hire's first mini performance appraisal. During this meeting you should review what the employee is excelling at and what they still require more improvement upon. Additionally, talk about goals for the employee that will inspire their continued professional development with your practice.

New Employee 1 Year Anniversary – The new hire is officially a full employee and it is time to celebrate! During the first-year anniversary this is the time to complete a thorough review of the employee's job description and determine where improvements can continually be made throughout this employee's continual career with your practice. This is also the time where you can discuss continued goals and where the employee falls on the overall pay structure for an employee in this specific role within the practice.

Throughout these phases, the most crucial factor that you can remember is to continually link every action back to the mission, vision, core values, and culture of your practice. You will find that the more often you can link your "why" to the different actions that are taking place within your office, the more effective your communication strategies will be and the more integrated into the culture your whole team will become.

Since she is beginning from nothing, Dr. Tooth realized that it is vital to remember that it is easier to develop a culture than it is to change a culture in the future. When you develop and maintain your culture in your ideal form, you will be able to uphold its prevalence within your practice throughout all your actions and the actions of your team. However, without proper and continual management, your culture becomes prone to shape shifting into something you did not intend it to be as it is continually affected by the experiences and actions that your entire team brings into the practice daily. Throughout this entire process, Dr. Tooth has come to understand the importance of having a strong and effective performance management system to uphold the desired culture of her practice.

Performance Management Systems – Because Consistency Mitigates the Risk of Complaints

Now that you have your team in place it is time to focus on the daily, weekly, monthly, and annual personnel management meetings that were broadly outlined within the onboarding process. While onboarding focuses on the first year of an employee's career within your practice, performance management requirements do not vanish after an employee's first year of employment is complete.

Dr. Tooth now has a team of four employees that are helping her to grow the practice of her dreams. Now that the practice has been open for six months the team is starting to find a good flow of working with one another. However, the growth that they once saw consistently has halted and that novel excitement that was once sizzling hot within the practice has cooled to a simmer. Dr. Tooth knows that there is more room for growth at the practice. She has big plans and goals for hiring more doctors, other employees and eventually opening a second location in a nearby neighborhood. How can she reenergize her team in a way that will give her the results that she is looking for, within the timeline that she desires?

Dr. Tooth is yet again in another situation where the ball is in her court to determine how fast the practice will grow and how to inspire that intrinsic motivation or 'internal drive' within her team that they once had before. The first thing that Dr. Tooth should do is look at her performance management system. Is Dr. Tooth relying on annual performance appraisals and goal setting sessions and hoping that this will be enough to continue that upwards momentum that the team once had? It is likely, based on the amount of growth that she hopes to continue to maintain, that relying on once per year performance metrics will not be enough to support her goals. Dr. Tooth should consider implementing a spectrum of daily, weekly, and monthly goals to supplement the annual performance goals that are already scheduled to take place.

Daily management goals should be initiated at a basic level to maintain the culture of the practice and keep up with small, achievable goals. These goals can include items such as daily production goals for administrators, same day treatment goals for assistants, and production per hour rates for hygiene team members. The goals should be somewhat easily obtainable on a daily basis. It is important to have goals that are just barely out of the reach of the employees so that they can feel that they need to stretch a bit to obtain them. However, these goals should not be so outlandish that they feel like they are impossible to obtain. This will also work to help your team to increase their overall employee morale within the workplace when they are achieving set goals every day.

Weekly management goals should be slightly more complex and a little more specific to individual departments. This might look like weekly production and A/R goals for your administrators, conversion rates based on case acceptance percentages for your assistants and specified reappointment rates for your hygiene team members. Again, there is continual benefit to having goals that are a bit of a stretch for your team members, but these must be goals that are not so out of reach that your team members do not even try to achieve them.

At the end of the week, you should debrief with your team and discuss the following:

What goals were met? How were they achieved? How can you increase this goal for next week?

What goals were not met? What got in the way of achieving these goals? How can you improve your results next week?

What will you focus on achieving next week?

Monthly management goals will be yet again more comprehensive than the daily and weekly goals set more frequently. For example, monthly goals may look like reaching $150,000 in monthly production for your administrators, reaching your 80% case acceptance rate for your assistants and producing $250/hour in the hygiene chair, having a reappointment rate of 85%, and selling 10 whitening treatments for your hygiene team members. For monthly goals to continue to uphold their momentum, it is important for the employees to understand why they should strive to hit these goals. There does not necessarily need to be external motivation provided so long as employees can see and understand why achieving these goals is important to the practice and then they can determine why reaching these goals is important to them on a personal level (research shows that an increase in external motivation techniques (for example: more $$) are correlated with a decrease in intrinsic motivation or internal drive).

Achievement can become habitual within the culture of a workplace, which makes it even more important to stay on top of these daily, weekly, and monthly goals. If departments have been meeting their goals for months at a time and then suddenly cease to try or care about achieving their goals, you need to look internally and determine what has drastically shifted the employee's perspective within the office. Is there some interpersonal conflict actively taking place? Did something happen to the employee outside of the office that is affecting their work capabilities? Is there something happening within the practice that is distracting an employee or diminishing their ability to hit their targets or goals?

Overall, the more that daily, weekly, and monthly department goals can be linked to individual role KPIs and KSAs, the more aligned they will be to support the annual performance appraisals that you conduct within your practice. Bonus points go to those employers that can also link their mission, vision, core values, and ideal culture back to the daily, weekly, and monthly goals set for their teams! Integrating all these concepts together is the perfect combination for the creation of a highly motivated and achievement-oriented team.

Finally, we have reached the crux of the performance management process – the individual, annual performance appraisal or 'employee review' as it is commonly named. This annual review usually covers:

- A review of the employees Job Description and any updated KPIs

- An observational skills assessment overview from the

    employee's immediate supervisor or manager

- Setting goals for the following year

- Potentially a salary review (not all practices desire to link pay with performance. If you do not wish to have pay linked with performance within your practice, do not couple a performance review with a salary increase, or you will have set a precedent that will indefinitely be an applicable standard within your office)

Again, because you are in the start-up phase, you truly have the power to set the stage of how all your performance appraisals are going to take place from this point forwards. Some practices get stuck, at the mercy of their employees, and are so afraid to conduct performance reviews because employees have come to expect an automatic raise included with their review, that they have completely stopped conducting annual employee reviews at all. This not only creates a huge disservice to the entire organization, but also changes the power dynamic within the employment relationship between the employee and the employer.

If there is one piece of HR related information that you take away from this chapter, we want it to be this:

Never allow yourself to be at the mercy of your employees.

This situation is characteristic of business owners who do not know or understand how to run a business, and therefore take as gospel any information that their employees provide to them (as long as the employee states it with enough conviction to be believable). We have seen these situations countless times as employer after employer is taken advantage of by their employees.

Stay knowledgeable and define your policies definitively from the very inception of your business opening and you will greatly mitigate the risk of ending up in this situation where you cannot even provide performance management coaching to your team without feeling like you are on the hook for providing an employee with a raise after the process is complete.

Off-boarding – Terminations, and Layoffs and Resignations, Oh My!

Dr. Tooth has been working hard with her team now for eighteen months! She can't believe the growth that she has seen from the team members and the goal setting strategies she is using consistently are working well within the practice. However, her newest hire isn't fitting in with the team or the culture of the practice all that well. She can tell after four months that this employee is likely just not a good fit for the organization and she thinks that she wants to go back to the recruitment phase and look for a different employee who will mesh with the team more cohesively. What should Dr. Tooth do now?

Termination is one of those tricky subjects that when completed correctly, can be a smooth transition process. However, terminations are often coupled with high levels of emotion and this can make high-level cognition a difficult process at times for both the employer and an employee. You have taken the best step possible by educating yourself more on this topic so that when it comes to terminating someone you are ready to take the best course of action.

Let's start with an overview of the variety of both voluntary and involuntary employee departures from a practice.

Termination Due to Performance – This is the type of termination that will follow the progressive discipline procedure (verbal warning ⏩ written warning ⏩ final written warning with suspension ⏩ termination due to performance). Clear documentation of the different warnings that were provided to the employee will be important in protecting the employer in the event of any legal proceedings that the former employee wishes to pursue.

<u>Termination Due to Misconduct</u> – This is the type of termination that generally follows a major incident (at the fault of the employee) within the workplace. Employers should do their due diligence with a proper investigation and interviews after an incident of this nature occurs and should document the findings for the employee's record before proceeding to terminate based on gross misconduct within the workplace. Ensure that you have evidence of the gross misconduct reported and documented to protect yourself in the event of any legal proceedings that the former employee wishes to pursue

<u>Termination Due to Ongoing Absenteeism</u> – This is the type of termination that generally follows when an employee does not show up to work for at least three consecutive days and where the employee cannot be reached to discuss why they are not at work. It is important to note that this type of termination should be processed through registered mail so that you have acknowledgement that the employee did actually receive the termination notice in the mail.

<u>Termination at No Fault of the Employee/Layoff/Reduction in Force</u> – This is the type of termination that takes place when an organization needs to restructure, or if a job or role within the practice becomes redundant. In this case, the employee has not done anything specific to warrant their termination, the organization just simply does not have the means to support an individual in this role anymore. Before terminating an employee due to organizational restructuring or job redundancy, it is best practice to determine if this employee could be trained in another department or role within the practice so that they can provide more value to the organization and stay continuously employed. This may or may not be applicable to your individual situation if you ever end up in a circumstance where you need to lay off employees. It is important in this situation to ensure that you are not immediately hiring anyone in this same role, or you will open yourself up to potential complaints from your previous employee to the US Department of Labour, as well as the potential for the laid off employee to pursue legal action against you for wrongful dismissal. Ensure that you also provide these employees with fantastic reference letters in order to help them secure future employment more easily.

<u>Furlough</u> – This is a temporary layoff of employment. When employees are furloughed, they must be provided with some additional information including: reasonable notice of the furlough taking place, when the furlough will begin and when the employee will be reinstated at work, why furlough is the only reasonable option for the employee and how employees will be notified of any changes to their status during this time of temporary layoff. Additionally, if you have

any salaried-exempt employees, please note your state and any contractual requirements for pay during a period of furlough.

Resignation – This is a type of voluntary termination where the employee is choosing to leave the practice on their own volition. Upon receipt of a resignation notice, it is best practice to provide the employee with a letter of acceptance of their resignation that stipulates all the details of their PTO, Benefits, Banked Overtime, and when their Final Compensation will be paid to them. As well, this notice should also notify them of any company equipment or property that they need to return to the practice, any access codes or passwords that will need to be disclosed, when they will need to provide this property or information to the practice, and the date when their exit interview will take place to determine why they have chosen to leave the practice. Ensure that you also provide these employees with fantastic reference letters to help them secure future employment more easily.

Now you must ask yourself, what are your obligations as an employer when you terminate an employee?

1. Know Your Legislation – your state legislation is going to provide you with the most up to date information regarding any legal requirements to your employees

2. Know Your Best Practice – sometimes it is not enough to just follow the legal minimum requirements. This is especially the case when other offices in your region are consistently providing more than just the legal minimum when off-boarding employees

3. Protect Your Privacy – it is vital to ensure that your terminated employees do not have access to any private or confidential materials once they are no longer employed by you. Make sure that they don't have any remote access to any files, documents, emails, or servers once they are no longer employed by you

4. Get in Front of Your Problems – if you have a suspicion that a former employee is going to take legal action against you due to something that has happened in the workplace, talk to an employment lawyer **_PRIOR_** to initiating the termination process. Your employment lawyer will be able to guide you through the best course of action to mitigate the risk of an employee being able to sue you in the future. This is the biggest example of not tripping over the $100 bill while you are scrambling to pick up the $5 bill. Investing in professional services when you think you need them

preemptively will be a huge cost saving (and stress reducer) in the long term.

Now that you have a high-level overview of terminations, layoffs and resignations, what should Dr. Tooth do?

A) Nothing – Dr. Tooth should have terminated this employee during the probationary period and now that this employee has progressed past the probationary period Dr. Tooth is stuck with her. Maybe if the team knows how much Dr. Tooth doesn't like this employee, they can pass the message along and the employee will resign?

B) Reduce the employee's hours so that they get the hint that they are not welcome in the practice and hope that they resign on their own accord.

C) Terminate – because the employee has only been with the practice for four months there is no obligation for severance or termination pay. Cut your losses quickly and move on to the next employee.

D) Terminate, but understand the requirements that are due to the employee prior to starting the termination process. Read your state laws regarding termination and/or severance pay requirements before preparing a severance package to terminate. Ensure that you ask yourself the following questions when developing a severance package: Do you want to have a full and final release signed so that the employee cannot sue you for wrongful termination? How old is the employee? Are they within any protected classes? Do you have insurance requirements (20+ employees, related to the Consolidated Omnibus Budget Reconciliation Act - COBRA)? How difficult will it be for this employee to find a job at another office in your region?

Answer:

D. While you might not be required to provide a severance package (unless it is stipulated in your offer letter or employment agreement that you will provide one), it is becoming more common that the best employers to work for in the USA are providing some kind of severance package to assist employees in their transition from one job to the next when they are not terminated for reasons based on their own actions.

At the time of this writing, the Fair Labour Standards Act (FLSA) does not require that base severance be paid to any employee in any workplace of any size.

The Not-So Good, the Bad, and the Ugliest – Why HR Always Deserves a Seat at the Table

Every small business owner starts their company with a dream. Besides dedicated HR companies, the dream of most small business owners is not to be an HR pro. However, regardless of whether you want to own and operate one small office with ten staff members, or you want to grow your brand to twenty offices and two hundred employees, the importance of HR within your practices does not change. HR will always deserve a seat at the table.

The previous information has been provided to you with the hopes that you are able to always mitigate the risk of having major problems with your staff. Unfortunately, most major problems with employees end up in mediation, arbitration or in court – in other words, they are expensive to manage when operate with a reactive HR model If you take the advice provided here regarding clear communication, mutual expectations, and solid management of the employee lifecycle, you will be able to be a proactive and confident employer that your team will quickly learn to know and trust.

To conclude, here is a mini cheat sheet of items to consider as you recruit, manage, and terminate your team over decades of success within the practice of your dreams:

- Stay up to date on your federal, state, and municipal employment legislation

- Understand how Human Rights legislation intersects with employment standards

- Ensure that you stay up to date with your OSHA compliance standards, including annual reporting and training requirements and that your OSHA documentation supports the information in your Infection Prevention Program and Manual.

- Keep your employee files tidy – know and understand how to fill out and file your I-9s and when other items become inactive within an employee file

- Ensure that your employees are classified correctly (for example: W-2 vs 1099)

- Keep good records of employee complaints and grievances, and ensure that you investigate, interview, and follow up as required

- Systemize your progressive discipline model to reduce claims of unfair treatment

- Know your rights as an employer when it comes to pre-employment, random and reasonable suspicion drug testing

- Have your emergency procedures playbook and training ready to implement right from your first day so that your team is confident in how to respond to an emergency. Empowered teams **respond,** untrained teams **react.**

- Have your vaccination policy ready, as well as a plan of action for how you will handle the situation if an employee cannot receive a highly recommended vaccine due to a protected reason

- Know your requirements as an employer regarding protected leaves, vacation days, holiday pay, sick days, and minimum wage requirements

Overall, we hope that we have made the message clear that you need strong and clear policies and procedures in place (and in writing) so that you can give the practice of your dreams the best start possible. Your policies and procedures are not expected to be written in stone, and realistically, they *should* change over time because the entire employment landscape changes over time. Legislation changes, best practice changes, your team will change, new ways of operating will become the norm, and realistically your HR program should have a full review annually to ensure that it is as effective as possible. Do not be scared if in ten years you look at your employee handbook and it looks entirely different from the one that you started with – that should be expected!

Remember, compliance is easy to maintain if you never fall out of line. You have the opportunity to start your practice as a 100% compliant employer. This is much easier than taking a pre-existing practice that is severely out of compliance and attempting to retroactively undo all the damage that has been done to build it back up to the 100% mark. You can start off perfectly – give yourself and your practice the best chance for victory by setting up your team for continued success from the very first new hire!

Chapter 9

Insurance and PPO Participation

By Michael Ingram

Insurance & PPO Participation

INTRODUCTION

The dental insurance market is complex, confusing, and constantly changing. In this chapter we're going to look at some common insurance company practices, how they affect your revenue and profitability, and how you can make the most of working with insurance plans and PPOs. Also included at the end of the chapter is a glossary of acronyms, terms, and definitions.

As a start up dental practice, the dentist faces decisions from practice location, size, name, staffing, marketing, financing, and countless others. One of those decisions will be how to attract and retain patients. In today's world, most dentists feel the need to join insurance plans and PPOs as their primary means of growth. This is very logical as over many years patients have been conditioned to select in network providers. In most cases, the insurance company will offer incentives through the benefit plan, to direct patients to in network dentists.

Through benefit design, payment protocols and other administrative hurdles, the insurance companies can make it difficult on out of network providers as they try to force you into a contract. And since many insurance companies will not negotiate fee schedules, you're left with "take it or leave it" schedules that require significant discounts from your practice fees. The dentist must decide to either stay out of network, and risk not being able to attract and retain patients, or accepting very low fee schedules in return for being listed as in network. Neither is an attractive offer, but in the end most dentist decide to join the insurance plans and PPOs.

PROBLEMS WORKING WITH INSURANCE & PPOS

Dental insurance is unique in a number of ways, but the most impactful way is through "Network Sharing Arrangements". Network sharing works like this

- You sign a contract with Insurance ABC, expecting to be "in network" for Insurance ABC patients.

- You later find out that the contract and fee schedule are also being used by Insurance XYZ and Insurance 123.

- Whether you like it or not, you are now in network for these additional insurances, and they are using the ABC's fee schedule to pay claims.

- When you continue to add more direct insurance contracts, the Network Sharing continues and grows, creating more in network situations with even more insurances.

Network Sharing can benefit a practice if done correctly and monitored closely, but most practices are not even aware the sharing is taking place. A situation where sharing can work is

- Insurance ABC has a reasonable fee schedule you can accept.

- Insurance ABC shares their fee schedule with Insurance XYZ and Insurance 123.

- By contracting with ABC, you are now in network for patients of ABC, XYZ and 123 at a single fee schedule that is acceptable.

- Instead of needing three contracts to be in network, you now only have one.

Unfortunately, dental insurance companies don't make it this easy and situations like the above example are rare. Most insurances share with multiple other insurances, and they also add Umbrella PPOs, which makes it extremely difficult for the practice to monitor all the relationships and who is using what fee schedule. Overall, Network Sharing arrangements create more problems than they solve for the practice.

The bigger problem with Network Sharing is that it leads to "Payment Downgrading", which is where the insurance plan will use the lowest fee schedule available to pay a claim. They "cherry pick" the lowest rate available, which leads to reduced revenue and makes payments less predictable, leading to other administrative issues. Let's look at another example

Dr. Smith has direct contracts with most all the major dental insurance companies as well as an Umbrella PPO.

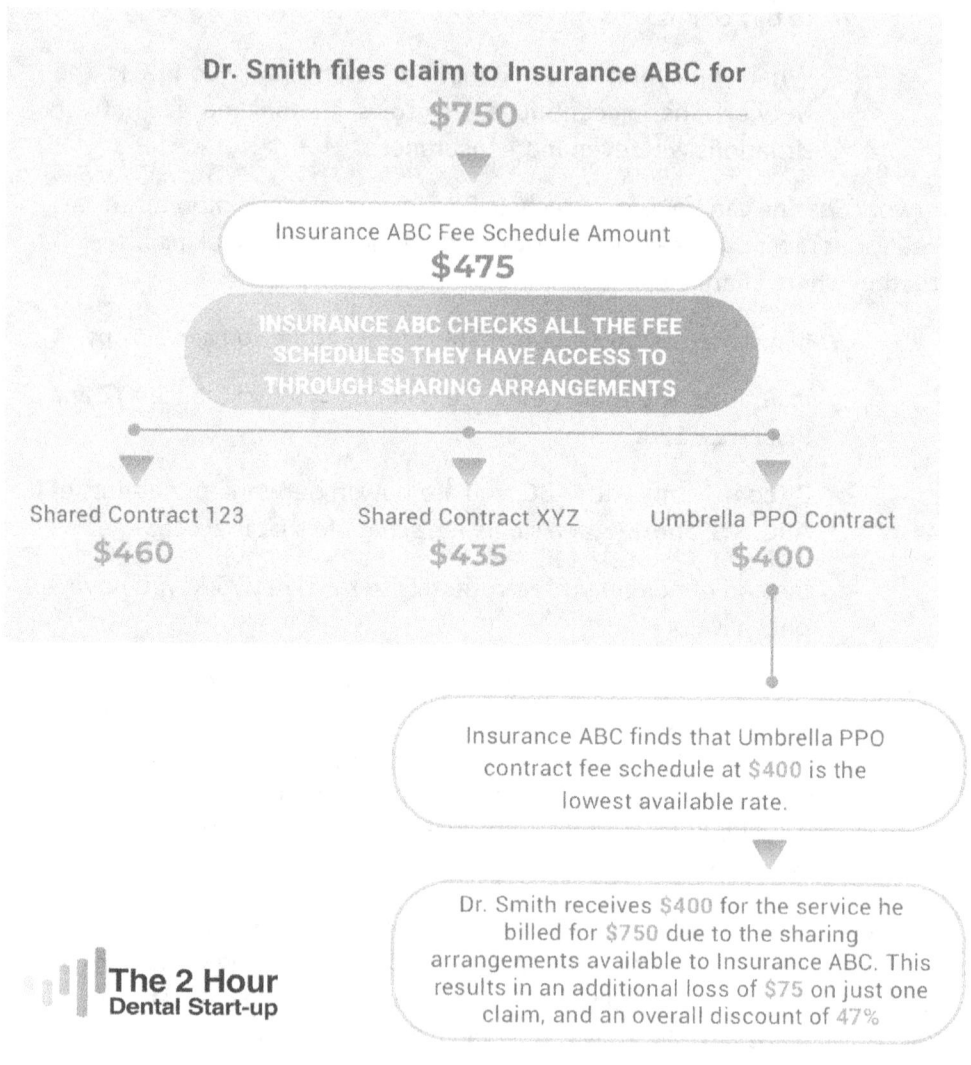

Dr. Smith files claim to Insurance ABC for
$750

Insurance ABC Fee Schedule Amount
$475

INSURANCE ABC CHECKS ALL THE FEE SCHEDULES THEY HAVE ACCESS TO THROUGH SHARING ARRANGEMENTS

Shared Contract 123
$460

Shared Contract XYZ
$435

Umbrella PPO Contract
$400

Insurance ABC finds that Umbrella PPO contract fee schedule at $400 is the lowest available rate.

Dr. Smith receives $400 for the service he billed for $750 due to the sharing arrangements available to Insurance ABC. This results in an additional loss of $75 on just one claim, and an overall discount of 47%

The 2 Hour
Dental Start-up

You're probably asking how this can be legal, but rest assured it is completely legal and Payment Downgrading happens all the time for a practice with multiple insurance and PPO contracts.

Another item to consider is how contracting with multiple insurance plans and PPOs will impact the operational and administrative aspects of your practice. For every insurance plan there is a contract that must be signed and a credentialing application that must be completed (and recertified every 2-3 years). For every insurance contract there is a fee schedule that must be loaded and kept updated. For every insurance or PPO, there is a client list that must be monitored as it constantly changes. Treatment plans must be calculated based on which fee schedule you think will be used, but once payment is made you must recalculate because they used a different schedule to pay. You may have to issue refunds, or collect additional payments from the patient, all while trying to get through the day-to-day requirements of running a dental practice.

STRATEGIES AND SOLUTIONS

Now that we've reviewed some of the pitfalls and problems with contracting multiple insurance plans and PPOs, let's look at some alternative strategies and solutions. I'll start by saying that all dental practices are unique, no two are alike regardless of type, location or even contracting strategy. However, we've developed basic strategies and rules that can help most practices achieve the growth they need while receiving reimbursement that is acceptable.

It goes without saying that if you can be a successful Fee for Service practice, that is the best situation. While you may file claims for your patients, ultimately you can balance bill and collect your full fees. You are not held captive by the insurance company discounts and other hassles that cause additional work and add cost to every patient. Unfortunately, today most new start-ups are not able to be fee for service, so we need to find a way to create a successful practice while also minimizing the impact insurance plans and PPO discounts have on the practice.

Before you start the contracting process, you should outline specific goals and work your strategy to achieve the goals.

DEVELOP A GOAL

- MINIMIZE the number of insurance contracts

- MINIMIZE the discounts taken by the contracts

- MAXIMIZE the number of insurance plans where you are in network

STRATEGY QUESTIONS

- How does the contracted fee schedule compare to my practice fees, and other insurance and PPO contracts (what's the effective discount)?

- Who, other than the insurance company you are contracting with, has access to the fee schedule (who are they sharing with)?

- Am I able to get this same insurance or patients through another contract (existing or otherwise), and how do those fee schedules compare?

- Can I afford to give up 45%+ in discounts just to attract new patients. Keep in mind that at discounts like these, you are seeing every third patient for free.

- Are they're experts that can help or alternatives that you should explore.

Once you have a goal and develop a strategy, you can take logical and intentional steps to reach the goal. Keep in mind there is no perfect solution, but choices you must make to arrive at the solution that works best for your practice situation.

One set of guidelines we recommend is to have no more than five total contracts. This typically consists of

- One Umbrella PPO (the one with the best fee schedule and most extensive client list).

- Mission critical contracts- those insurances that are so large in the market you feel the need to be in network since they have so many members (patients) in your area. In a lot of areas that can be Blue Cross (BCBS) or Delta Dental, but they may vary in your market.

- BCBS, Delta and Cigna are not often available through other sharing or Umbrella PPOs, so they usually require direct contracts.

The benefits of this contracting strategy are several. First, you have a minimal number of contracts attached to the practice. Second, the Umbrella PPO will likely give you access to most of the insurance plans other than BCBS, Delta, Cigna. Third, BCBS, Delta and Cigna don't share with other insurances, and for the most part don't use Umbrella's, so network sharing and payment downgrading are kept to a minimum, if not eliminated entirely.

However, there can be downsides such as extremely low fee schedules. You need to balance your patient base as much as possible, meaning don't let one insurance become too dominant in your practice. Umbrella PPOs often have better fee schedules and allow some degree of negotiating, but the discounts may still be significant. Not all insurance plans may be included in the Umbrella PPO networks. For example, regular commercial insurance patients may be covered, but those in Federal or Military plans may be excluded.

Another item I'll touch on briefly is the importance of offering a practice membership plan. These plans will allow you to offer "cash patients" a way to prepay for their dental care versus paying all at once. You are able to select the services that are included as well as the price for the membership plan, which is usually offered either as a monthly or annual amount. Membership plans are proven to create loyalty to your practice and treatment acceptance is often higher for plan members. These plans help create a steady cash flow for the practice and provide other financial benefits as well. There are a number of companies that specialize in practice membership plans, and you should have this on your list of options to explore as you prepare to open your office.

CREDENTIALING AND ENROLLMENT PROCESS

Once you've developed your primary goal and strategy, it's time start the process of contracting, credentialing, and enrollment. It is important to realize that this is a lengthy and time-consuming process, that often takes months to complete. You will want to start this process as early as possible before opening your practice, but keep in mind that the insurances will not credential you until all the required information and documents are available. For example, if you don't have your liability insurance in place, you will not be allowed through the credentialing process. This creates a situation where you can't get started as early as you might like, but it's important to start as early as you can. Just know that you will likely not be fully enrolled in all the insurance plans when you open your doors.

You will need to contact the individual insurance companies and Umbrella PPOs, requesting a contracting packet, fee schedule and client list. Once you have these in hand, you should create a spreadsheet that shows your practice fees and the top 25-30 codes you bill and include all fee schedules for each insurance and PPO for comparison. You may realize that the discounts required are too much to accept, and you may also identify others that have better schedules than you expected. You should also speak to the contracting representative at the insurance company or Umbrella PPO and ask specific questions about network sharing arrangements and how long credentialing and enrollment will take once you return the application. Once you have all this information you can see how the insurances overlap, where sharing occurs, and other valuable information that allows you to confirm your overall strategy.

Now that you've confirmed your strategy and the list of insurances and PPOs to contract with, you'll need to sign the contracts and complete the credentialing applications. Most credentialing applications ask for all the same information, but it's a time-consuming process, nonetheless. You should return the applications as you complete them, and you may want to prioritize the most important insurances and do them first. It's helpful to have all the required documents on hand when you start, here's a sample checklist.

- Contract/Participation Agreement

- Credentialing Application

- W-9

- Current Dental License

- Current DEA License

- Proof of Professional Liability Insurance

Other items may be required such as

- Current CDS/CSR

- Anesthesia/Sedation License/Permit

- Residency/Fellowship/Internship Certificates

- Proof of any specialty training

-

Credentialing and Enrollment are not the same thing but are connected. Once you return the application and contract, the process will work similar to the following.

- Insurance company receives your application and enters it into the "queue".

- Insurance will determine if they want to accept your application- this can be based on provider saturation in the market, or other factors, however most applications are accepted.

- The insurance company will submit your application to the credentialing committee- usually a group within the company that includes both clinical and non-clinical personnel. The point of the credentialing committee is to confirm your credentials meet their minimum requirements for network participation.

- Once you are approved by the committee, your application will be submitted to the enrollment department. Yes, you are now in yet another queue.

- Depending on the insurance company, your enrollment- the act of adding you to their network and entering your demographic file in their claims system- may takes days or even months. Some insurances do this in-house, but others may subcontract the process to a company in another country. While an insurance may tell you the status of your enrollment, there is little you can do to speed up the process.

- For Umbrella PPOs, the process is very similar, but the credentialing committee is part of the Umbrella. Following the approval of the committee, your demographic file is sent to the various insurances that use the PPO. From there, the enrollment process with the insurances is mostly the same.

You'll want to have a designated person and process for following up and tracking your enrollment progress. The effective date assigned to your contract will impact claims payments and you will want to confirm your listing on the insurance provider directory website. You are also now able to officially market yourself as a participating network provider for that insurance or PPO.

HOW TO GET HELP

Most dentist do not choose the field because they wanted to become business owners or contracting experts. Just as you would hire a CPA to help with your taxes, it's probably a good idea to consult an expert that can help with your insurance contracts. As with any industry, there is no shortage of "experts" that will help with the contracting process but be sure to speak with several and work with the one that focuses on doing what's best for your practice, not his or her bank account. If the consultant wants to be paid based on the number of contracts they do, find another consultant. If the consultant promises to "negotiate" all your contracts, be wary since so many insurances don't really negotiate. You might be paying for a fee schedule you could get yourself just by asking. If the consultant promises to give you all that you want, but the contract includes a lot of caveats and exclusions, and no guarantees, again you might want to keep looking. There are reputable consultants that will always put your interests first, but you may have to do some homework to find them.

Summary

The insurance and PPO world is complex, confusing, and constantly evolving, creating new ways to benefit the insurance company at the expense of the dentist. Deciding to join these plans is not something to be done without careful thought, research, having a process in place, patience and knowing that there is no perfect solution. I hope this information is a useful guide to help you navigate the difficult and confusing process of working with insurances and PPOs.

Acronyms, Terms & Definitions

Balance Billing: Charging the patient the difference between what their insurance allows and the dentist standard fees. This only applies if the dentist is out of network (OON) and not a member of the PPO.

Benefit Plan: The terms of the insurance plan that govern everything from what is covered, the amounts covered, exclusions, etc., even down to the paperwork that must be submitted for approval. Each insurance company can have dozens of Benefit Plans they administer.

Direct Contract: The signed agreement between the dentist and the insurance company to be a network provider at the designated reduced rate. The dentist is then referred to as being "In Network" (INN).

Credentialing: The process of verifying the dentists' credentials- education, malpractice history, etc.- to confirm they meet the credentialing standards of the insurance company or PPO.

Discount: This is the amount the dentist agrees to "write off" or discount his/her charges for being in-network. The contracted fee schedule will result in an average discount off the standard practice fees.

Enrollment: The process of an insurance company or PPO accepting and adding the dentist to their network and data management/claim system. As part of enrollment, the insurance will assign an effective date and start paying claims per the contract.

EOB: Explanation of Benefits. This is a statement that accompanies payment for a dental service. The EOB will also explain the payments, discounts and PPO/fee schedule utilized.

Fee For Service: A type of dental practice that is paid for 100% of its standard practice fees, either by a patient's insurance, cash, a finance plan, or a combination.

Fee Schedule: the list of codes and fees that the dentist agrees to accept as the maximum allowable reimbursement when signing a contract with an insurance plan or PPO.

Insurance Company: A company that sells dental insurance policies to individuals and companies, collects premiums, and pays claims. They may also have a network of directly contracted dentists and/or use Umbrella PPOs.

Network Sharing/Leasing: A mechanism by which an insurance or PPO shares its network of dentists with other insurances and PPOs, such that the first PPOs in-network dentists must then accept patients as in-network providers of the other PPOs.

Out of Network (OON): A dentist who is not a member of a PPO and does not hold a direct contract but provides dental care for a plan member (patient) as an OON dentist.

Payment Downgrading: As a PPO member in a shared network situation, the dentist gets paid the lowest fee available for a provided service offered by the various insurances in the sharing arrangement.

Payer: another term for insurance company.

PPO: Preferred Provider Organization. A network of dental providers that have agreed (signed contracts) to provide dental care to plan members at a certain discounted rate. The term PPO is also used to describe the networks associated with both direct contracts and umbrella networks.

Provider: Dentist/Dental practice.

UCR: Usual, Customary, & Reasonable. The amount paid for a dental service based on what providers in that area usually charge. The UCR is sometimes used to determine the allowed amount payable by the insurance company. The term can also be used to mean the standard fees charged by the practice.

Umbrella Network/PPO: A network or group of insurance companies under a single PPO contract. The Umbrella will offer access to their network to individual insurance companies as well as other PPOs, at the contracted fee schedule for the Umbrella.

About the Authors:

And how to get ahold of them

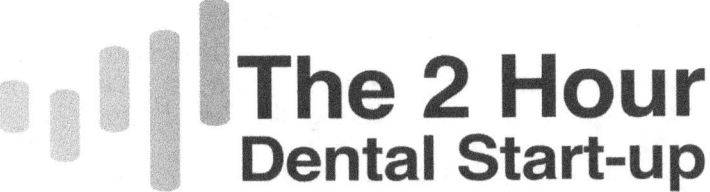

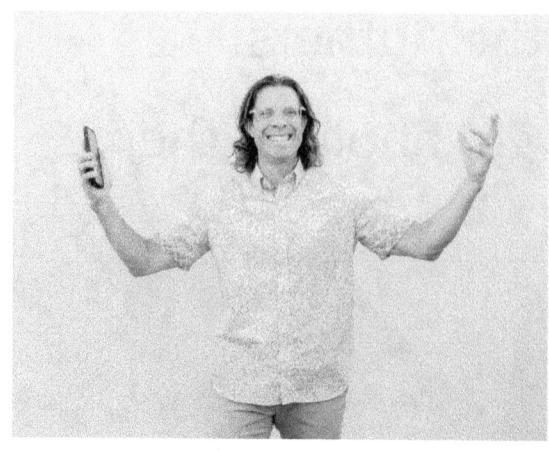

Eric Swarvar

Dental Industry

Extraordinaire

Since graduation from Stephan F. Austin State University in 2000, Eric has worked for only two companies, both in the dental industry. Located in Flower Mound, Texas

Eric has worked for a dental manufacturer and a dental supply company brining a unique experience serving his client base.

Eric not only specializes in dental start-ups, he also assists his currently client base in modernizing, updating, and adding technology to their practice for the benefit of their patients care.

When Eric is not dentaling, he enjoys being outside living an active lifestyle and spending time with his family. Eric also enjoys providing mentorship for college aged young adults and speaks annually at his alma mater's college of business.

Founder of the 2 Hour Dental Start-up

Founder of Dental Equipment Hacks YT Channel

Lover of people, coffee, and bikes

https://the2hourdentalstartup.com

eswarvar@gmail.com

www.linkedin.com/in/eric-swarvar

Jennifer Edwards
Dental Lender
Aficionado

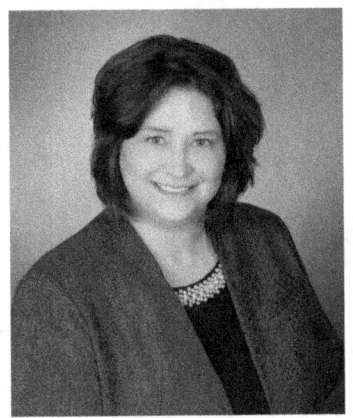

Jennifer has over 20 years of business lending and banking experience. Prior to joining Sunflower Bank, she also worked at Chase Bank, Wells Fargo and Regions Bank.

Sunflower Bank, N.A. is a regional community bank with approximately $4 billion in assets dedicated to building long-term relationships founded on sound principles and trust. We operate as Sunflower Bank, First National 1870 and Guardian Mortgage, working together to serve all of your business and personal banking needs.

jennifer.edwards@sunflowerbank.com

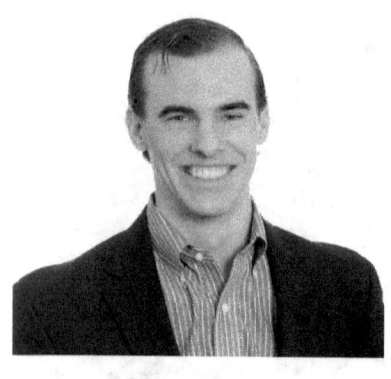

Peter Hays
Healthcare Real Estate Expert

Healthcare Real Estate, specializing in market and site selection for healthcare providers and medical professionals. My job is to ensure your real estate becomes an asset to your business and long-term goals by putting you into a location that will provide the best opportunity for success.

Practice Real Estate Group's proprietary research and analysis platform provides you with the most comprehensive data possible, combining industry-leading demographics and competition reports with the largest database of medical real estate listings. Utilizing our partnership-based business model, I build long-term relationships with clients based on trust and results.

My individual responsibilities include:

o   Creating and executing real estate strategies to implement client's business and investment goals.
o   Negotiating lease (Letter of Intent) and purchase (Letter of Offer) proposals, contracts on behalf of clients.
o   Providing in depth demographic studies, analysis of current and future population statistics and competition ratios.
o   Providing new markets for medical groups and private practice startups.
o   Guiding clients through the step by step process of purchasing land, medical office buildings, retail centers and owner occupy/ rent replacement opportunities.
o   Developing medical office projects in existing and new markets.

https://www.linkedin.com/in/peter-james-hays-ii-healthcare-real-estate-expert-715428125/

phays@practicerealestategroup.com

Erick Cutler is the

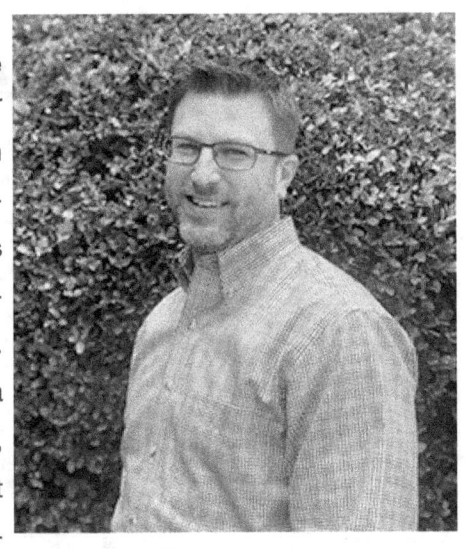

partner-in-charge of the firm's Eisner Amper's Dental Group, focusing on the individual, group, and multi-location dental practices. He also works with individual dentists on their personal tax and compliance issues. Erick prides himself on taking a holistic approach to client service, which includes practice management and consulting, business and practice strategies, tax planning and compliance, and consulting on the overall financial health of the practice and the practice owners. With the goal of best serving his clients, he brings new and innovative ideas and strategies to the table and makes sure the owners maintain an awareness and understanding of their practice's financial health.

214.252.7917
Erick.Cutler@EisnerAmper.com
https://www.linkedin.com/in/erick-cutler-8a40ab9/

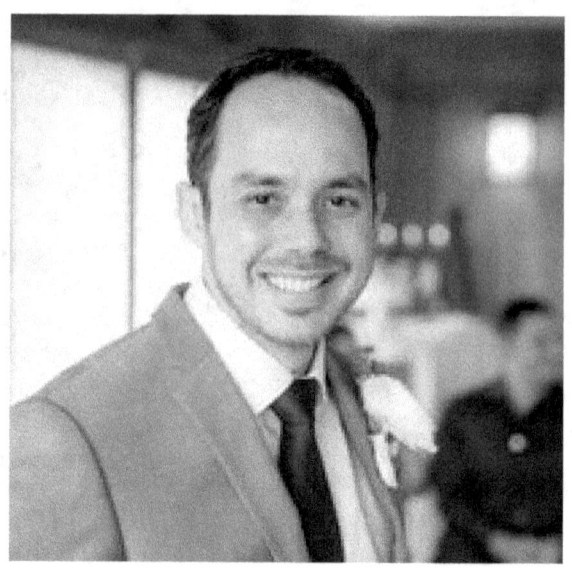

William Cruz
Dental Office Design Guru

Having graduated with an architectural degree from the University of Texas at Arlington, I always hoped that I would get a chance to help people build their dream space, and fortunately for me, at Midwest Dental, we can do exactly that. Being a smaller company, we can offer a boutique service that doctors would not be able to get with larger dealers; we can sit and have one-on-one conversations and discuss the design in a very detailed and interactive manner. At the end of the day, the design ends up being the fruit of a very collective work.

Some of my academic/professional accomplishments:
• Graduated Cum Laude with a Bachelor's degree in Political Science from the University of North Texas
• Graduated Magna Cum Laude with a Bachelor's degree in Architecture from the University of Texas at Arlington
• Graduated Magna Cum Laude with a Master's degree in Structural Engineering from the University of Texas at Arlington
• Member of National Honors Societies
• Fluent in the latest 3D building design software

Some of my hobbies and interests:
• Hang out with friends and watch a good movie
• Travel to interesting places
• Have a glass of wine while having a good conversation
william.cruz@midwestdental.com
https://www.linkedin.com/in/william-cruz-aa752572/

Michael T. Ingram
Vice President, Business Development
Dental Advocacy Group

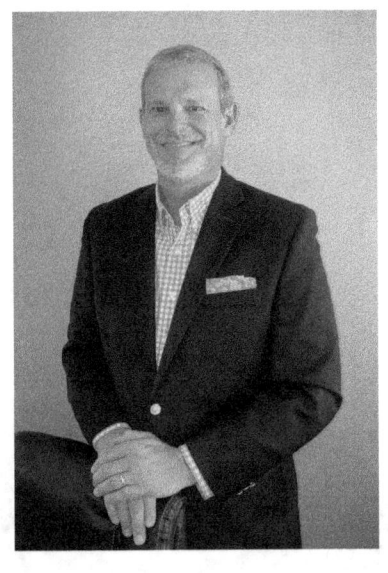

After receiving my degree from the University of North Alabama, I've been in the insurance and healthcare space for over 27 years. I've worked for a diverse group- from a fortune 500 hospital company to a start-up medical PPO, to a national ancillary care network. Four years ago, I joined Dental Advocacy Group with goal of growing the company through our unique services, and by developing strategic partnerships with like-minded dental organizations and industry experts. Over this time, we've been fortunate to partner with companies like Midwest Dental, where our programs can help their clients increase practice revenue and profitability.

My role with Dental Advocacy Group allows me to draw on years of experience in business and relationship development. By focusing on key partner relationships, we can offer programs that truly increase revenue, while simplifying the insurance and PPO contracting process. By working directly with our partners and clients, we develop and promote solutions that provide tangible, lasting value to the private dental practice.

Michael T. Ingram
(256) 701-0996
mingram@dentaladvocacygroup.com
www.dentaladvocacygroup.com

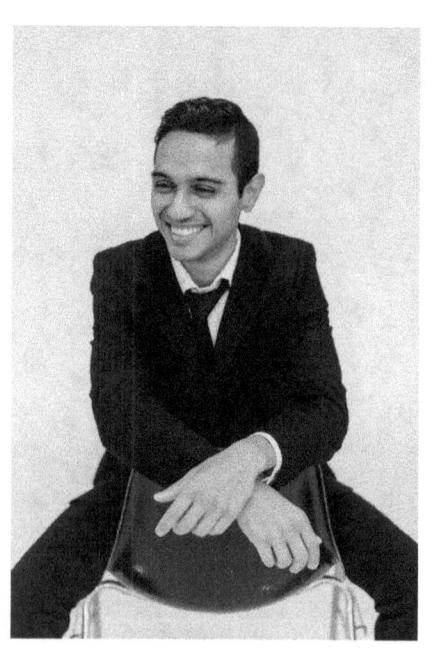

Michael Arias
The Dental Marketer

Have you ever looked around your community and thought to yourself...

I wonder how I can get the employees from Starbucks to come into our practice... or if only I can get those teachers from that school to come into my practice then that would be perfect! Maybe you've looked around your community and asked yourself: How can I get the members from that gym, the residents from those apartments, the employees from that corporation, to come into my practice and become my patient?

If you've EVER wondered or asked yourself that... then you are not alone. The great news is there is a solution for you. And you can do it all with no budget and no extra expenses.

In fact, this guy wants you to do this with a ZERO DOLLAR BUDGET!

If you've heard of Ground Marketing, then you've probably heard of the guy who coined that term: Michael Arias

Michael Arias teaches you exactly that.

He has been Ground Marketing for a little under a decade now and has mastered the way to get new patients from schools, clinics, day cares, senior homes, small business, banks, gyms, spas, restaurants and more locations all around your community!

- *The host/ founder of The Dental Marketer Podcast*

- *Creator of the only Ground Marketing Course in the world!*

- *Co-Founder of The Making of A Dental Start-Up*

- *Co-Founder of the only Pediatric Dental Marketing Course.*

You can read, see and hear him on The Dental Marketer Podcast or www.thedentalmarketer.org.

Olivia is an accomplished HR professional who brings over 12 years of direct business experience to the table when serving her clients. She holds multiple designations including the Chartered Professional in Human Resources (CPHR), Society of Human Resource Management Senior Certified Professional (SHRM-SCP) and most recently has obtained her Global Professional in Human Resources (GPHR) credential. Olivia is a self-proclaimed life-long learner and is presently completing her PhD in Industrial and Organizational Psychology.

Samantha Leonard has been in the Dental industry for over a dozen years. She has worked every role, worn every hat and mastered all the traits that eventually lead her to become an Operational Manager with a well-respected and world-renowned orthodontist, Dr. Sam Daher. Together, they started and built a multi-million-dollar practice from scratch and expanded to 6 locations across the country. Her managerial experience has helped her appreciate and identify the negative effect of a wrong hire, lack of systems and the adverse impact on team dynamic, quality of customer service, lost time and wasted money.

https://streamdentalhr.com